## ACCLAIM FOR
*SMART QUESTIONS TO ASK YOUR DOCTOR*

"That the patient be well-informed is a necessity for health care decision making in the 1990s. This book starts us down the path to that necessary information by inaugurating the first step: asking smart questions!"

> —Bernard Adelsberg, M.D., Chief,
> Allergy and Immunology, Nassau
> County Medical Center, New York

"Written with the insight of a practicing physician, the book answers the important questions that all consumers must address when using the health care system . . . SMART QUESTIONS TO ASK YOUR DOCTOR makes every medical consumer an equal partner with their health care practitioner."

> —Charles B. Inlander, President,
> People's Medical Society

"A thorough and complete compilation . . . Extremely valuable to anyone contemplating medical questions. By eliminating fear of the unknown and placing patients in control of their health, it shall improve an individual's chance of a complete and easy recovery."

> —Richard A. Bloch, Founder,
> Bloch Cancer Foundation

## Other books in the *Smart Questions* series

Smart Questions to Ask Your Doctor
Smart Questions to Ask Your Lawyer
Smart Questions to Ask Your Insurance Agent
Smart Questions to Ask Your Stockbroker
Smart Questions: Interview Your Way to Job Success

## Published by
## HarperPaperbacks

# SMART QUESTIONS TO ASK YOUR DOCTOR

## DOROTHY LEEDS
### WITH JON M. STRAUSS, M.D.

HarperPaperbacks
*A Division of HarperCollinsPublishers*

HarperPaperbacks    *A Division of* HarperCollins*Publishers*
10 East 53rd Street, New York, N.Y. 10022

Cover design by Richard Rossiter

First printing: April 1992

Printed in the United States of America

HarperPaperbacks and colophon are trademarks of HarperCollins*Publishers*

10 9 8 7 6 5 4 3 2

This book is dedicated, with appreciation, to my literary agent Barbara Lowenstein. Without her help, belief, and perseverance, this book, and the ones that follow, would not have been.

# ACKNOWLEDGMENTS

Special thank-yous to:
Dr. Bernard Adelsberg, for his professional and loving advice.
Arthur Ashe, Richard A. Bloch, Dr. Helen De Rosis,
Charles Inlander, Mary Ann Liebert, and Stephanie
Simonton for their gracious endorsements.
Karen Solem, a great lady and a great editor.
Chris Wilhide, who was always there when we needed her.
Norman Kurz, for his excellence, kindness, and patience.
Robert Shook and Terrie Williams, the two greatest net-
workers in the world, who have generously shared so
much with me.

Dr. Strauss and I both want to express our appreciation
for Sharyn Kolberg, whose calm demeanor and excellent
writing skills make it all seem easy.

Dr. Strauss also says thank-you to:
Mollie Stevens, for her invaluable help and support.
Leroi Chittendom, for his patience and listening abilities.
Gloria Strauss, my mother, for teaching me to ask questions.
Jack Strauss, my father, who taught me to check out all
the answers.

# CONTENTS

# INTRODUCTION

When you are in need of medical attention, how do you choose the doctor best qualified to diagnose or treat your current problem? If a doctor prescribes medication for you, are you aware of all of its potential side effects? How do you know whether the surgery your physician has just recommended is absolutely necessary? You don't know unless you *ask questions*!

Often the need to ask questions is strongest when you are most vulnerable. When you are ill or in pain, you're likely to be frightened; you don't ask as many questions as you should. Consequently, you don't get the information you need.

For example, one young woman I know was diagnosed with an ovarian cyst. She was told to report to the hospital at 7:00 a.m. on Wednesday. She was so frightened that she didn't ask the doctor any questions—and when she got home, she couldn't remember any of his instructions. She went into the hospital on Wednesday, mentally prepared for surgery, only to find out that it was to be only a preliminary examination.

You may think that this young woman was an exception, that you would never act this way. Think again. My friend is an intelligent, successful attorney—but that didn't stop her from being frightened and intimidated by the whole experience. No matter how strong and resourceful you are in other areas of your life, you, too, probably respond to pain and illness with confusion and anxiety.

Yet this is often just the time when you are asked to make difficult decisions—decisions that may affect the rest of your life. Your health is your most important asset; you have the right, and the responsibility, to obtain information concerning your present and future well-being.

There is no need to let others assume control over your health, to allow anyone else to make decisions for you, or to feel that you are a victim of circumstance. This book was written to help you progress from being a victim to becoming a victor, and to show you how you can become a "questioning detective," uncovering the clues you need to make the best decisions. Become an educated patient and you become a healthier patient.

## INFORMATION OVERLOAD

We are now living in the age of information—and the fields of health and medicine are on information overflow. Our television sets and radios, as well as magazines and newspapers, assail our ears and eyes with health care messages. We can't eat our morning cereal or watch the evening news without being reminded of the virtues of losing weight, lowering cholesterol levels, or increasing fiber intake.

We are all bombarded with information—overloaded with facts, figures, advice, and opinions. The problem is that it's getting harder and harder to extract the information you really need. And when you find yourself in a situation where you need specific—and perhaps life-saving—information, all those facts, figures, advice, and opinions seem to fly right out the window. What can you do? How can you find out, right then and there, what you need to know?

You can ask questions.

## HOW I LEARNED THIS LESSON

Nine years ago, I was diagnosed with breast cancer. I was advised to have a mastectomy. At that time, almost everyone with breast cancer was given this advice. But I didn't believe that this was my only option. I was determined to find out whether there might be another way for me to stop my cancer and regain my health.

I started asking questions. I asked a lot of doctors a lot of questions. It was, at times, a very frustrating experience, because I really didn't know what I should be asking. There were many different theories and I heard varying opinions. Eventually, I was able to get enough information to enable me to make a logical, well-balanced decision. I found health care professionals who disagreed with my original doctor's advice or who felt that other treatments could be tried first. I decided on a lumpectomy, followed by radiation treatments and by a regime of diet and exercise to which I adhere to this day.

I learned a valuable lesson from this frightening experience: by asking questions, I gave myself options. I was able to make a decision that was best for me under the circumstances. This situation made me realize the importance of obtaining the information necessary on which to base an important medical decision.

There are only two ways to get that information. One is by watching and reading. For example, you might get some clues about a doctor's competence by observing the doctor's behavior in the office. You can probably read up on your illness and its possible treatments. This technique is fine for preparation and background information, but the only way to acquire immediate information, direct from the source's mouth and directly applicable to your own problem, is by asking questions.

## WHY DON'T WE ASK MORE?

The reason we don't ask more questions is largely because we are afraid to question authority. We follow the tradition that says, "The doctor knows best." We are afraid to doubt the doctor's advice.

We are reluctant to ask questions because:

- We don't want to offend the doctor.
- We assume that all doctors are competent just because they're doctors.
- We think we need medication, not information and explanations.

We are afraid to look stupid, afraid that by asking questions we will reveal our ignorance. The truth is just the opposite—we reveal our ignorance by blindly accepting the word of others.

## BUT WHAT DO I ASK?

Many times we don't ask questions because we are not sure what questions we should be asking. We tell ourselves that these people are the experts and should know what they are talking about. "The doctor should know what's wrong with me (and how to fix it); that's what he went to school for. He's the one who knows medicine. And besides, I DON'T EVEN KNOW WHAT QUESTIONS TO ASK."

We are faced with difficult decisions every time we go to a professional for medical attention, and often we come away with lingering doubts. "Was there something else I should have asked?" is the refrain that haunts most of us after we leave the doctor's office.

You might wish you had an expert to help you get at the facts that you require. Well, now you have. This book will turn *you* into the expert. Take it with you to the doctor's office. Or write down the questions that apply to your situation. For example, if you've been told that you should have surgery, concentrate on the section called "Smart Questions to Ask When You Need Surgery"; if you're looking for a doctor for your 3-year-old, read the section called "Smart Questions to Ask a Pediatrician."

Some of the questions are for you to ask yourself (for instance, when choosing a doctor, you may have to decide whether you prefer a man or a woman, whether a nonsmoking waiting room is important to you, or if you are able to travel to a doctor all the way across town). However, most of the questions are for you to ask the health professional.

Add your own questions to the list. I don't presume to have covered every possible medical situation. But the questions here should get you started and should stimulate your own questioning process so that you, too, can find out what you really need to know in order to make informed decisions.

## WHY YOU NEED THIS BOOK

The purpose of this book is threefold:

1. To provide you with the questions to ask in order to get the information you need.
2. To get you into the habit of asking questions.
3. To build your confidence in dealing with your doctor.

After all, the person who asks the questions sets the direction of the discussion and its topic and gains a sense of control in a difficult situation. Most psychologists agree that anxiety arises from loss of control. When you ask a question, the other person feels compelled to answer and the power goes to the asker. (Just watch the power shift when someone asks you, "Where are you going?" and you answer, "Why do you ask?")

You don't have to take the doctor's word for something just because he or she's a doctor or nod and say Yes if you don't understand. You don't have to leave the office until you get a satisfactory answer, no matter how intimidating the doctor may appear. You have the right to ask questions and the right to get answers. If a doctor won't answer your questions, get someone who will. If a doctor doesn't have time for explanations, there are other doctors around who are willing to provide them.

## A VERY WILLING DOCTOR

I was very fortunate, in writing this book, to have found a doctor who not only was willing and able to answer questions, but to ask them as well. Jon Strauss, M.D., is a general practitioner located in Berea, Kentucky. We share the same philosophy about medical care—that the patient and the doctor should establish a partnership. Doctors are human too, and may not always realize that they are intimidating or that a patient hasn't understood everything that's been said. Curing communications problems is one of the doctor's most important functions.

When I began talking to the medical community about this book, several doctors confided that they don't like patients who ask questions. They did not want to be confronted about their attitudes or abilities.

But I don't believe that all doctors share those feelings; Dr. Strauss is a perfect example.

I found communicating with Dr. Strauss easy and fun. He's nothing like the stereotypically intimidating authority figure we often imagine doctors to be. He's warm and sympathetic and has a wonderful sense of humor.

I chose Dr. Strauss for another reason, as well. All my experiences with doctors and hospitals have been in a large metropolitan area. I wanted to get another perspective, and I knew Dr. Strauss' rural practice would give him the perfect viewpoint in that regard.

Dr. Strauss and I don't claim to have exhausted all the questions you could, or should, ask your doctor. Nor do we intend to give you specific medical advice. Dr. Strauss has provided examples to give you a basis for comparison: when you ask a question, you may want to compare your doctor's answer with the one in the book.

**THE HE/SHE ISSUE**

One last word on a technical issue. We did not want to include any gender bias in this book by constantly using "he" to refer to the doctor. On the other hand, it is very awkward to use "he/she" and "him or her" throughout. So when referring to "the doctor," we use "he" in some examples and "she" in others.

**AND FINALLY . . .**

This is your opportunity to create a new relationship with your doctor and with your health. Become an active participant in your own medical care. Start asking smart questions. It could save your life.

# SECTION 1

## SMART QUESTIONS TO ASK BEFORE YOU SELECT A DOCTOR

For some people, selecting a doctor is like playing pin the tail on the donkey. They close their eyes, put a finger on a name in the telephone book, and hope that they have made a good choice.

Pin the tail on the donkey is a harmless children's game, but choosing a doctor is serious business. Your life may be at stake. There are many different types of doctors practicing in our country today, and you may not even know where to begin to find the particular kind of doctor you need. This section contains some general questions I asked Dr. Strauss in order to provide a basic understanding of how our medical system is set up.

\* \* \*

## WHY DO I NEED A DOCTOR?

There are two basic reasons why people go to the doctor:

1. For health maintenance
2. For problem solving and treatment

The reason you are seeking help can have a direct bearing on whom you choose to see. For example, if you have a specific ailment, such as a chronic digestive problem, you might want to see a gastroenterologist (a doctor who deals specifically, and exclusively, with digestive problems). On the other hand, if you are relatively healthy and want to make sure that you remain that way, you may want to see a primary care physician (such as a family practitioner) for a general checkup.

## IF I'M INTERESTED IN HEALTH MAINTENANCE, WHAT OPTIONS ARE AVAILABLE TO ME?

Believe it or not, there are almost as many different kinds of health care available as there are doctors from among whom to choose. There is the standard approach to health maintenance, under the guidelines of the American Medical Association (AMA), which includes annual physical examinations, Pap smears, mammograms, cholesterol reviews, etc. Then there are alternative health fields, and they have their own approaches toward health maintenance. Alternative methods include homeopathic vitamins (some health care professionals may recommend megadoses of vitamin C, A, B, or D, or herbs, such as chamomile and garlic); chiropractic manipulation (a system of healing which holds that disease results from a lack of normal nerve function and that employs spinal manipulation and adjustment to help you stay healthier); and reflexology (also called zone therapy, it is a specialized form of massage—usually of the hands or the feet—that allegedly is able to restore normality of function and to give relief from pain to virtually any part of the body).

## HOW DO I DECIDE WHAT KIND OF MAINTENANCE AND PREVENTION TO FOLLOW?

Preventative medicine and health maintenance are often a matter of personal preference and belief. If you are a traditional type of person, you may prefer to stick with conventional health care as established by the AMA. If you are more of a "back to nature" advocate, you may prefer alternative approaches to health maintenance.

Some people are willing to combine both forms. For example, a man with chronic back problems may consult both an orthopedic doctor (a bone specialist) and a chiropractor who specializes in holistic medicine (by considering the patient's health and life-style as a whole, rather than treating just one problem).

## HOW DO I CHOOSE WHAT'S RIGHT FOR ME?

The type of health maintenance you choose should match your overall life-style and beliefs. Ask your friends and family about their experiences (both positive and negative) with different kinds of health care maintenance. They may be able to recommend a certain field of medicine or a particular type of doctor. Then you can decide whether you want to follow their suggestions.

You can also do your own research. There is plenty of literature around, from popular scientific journals such as *Nature* and *Science* to general-interest magazines ranging from *Family Circle* to *Redbook* to *Prevention*. The ultimate decision, of course, rests on what feels best to you, based on your personal philosophy, your friends' and family's recommendations, your own research, and your basic common sense. In short, you have to decide what is right for you when it comes to staying healthy.

## HOW DO I FIND A DOCTOR WHO AGREES WITH MY IDEAS OF HEALTH MAINTENANCE?

The answer to this question is what this book is about: YOU'VE GOT TO ASK QUESTIONS. Ask your health care professional how he feels about medical practices—conventional or alternative. Find out what his medical philosophy is and see whether you agree with it.

The reason for asking a traditional doctor about alternative health care is to compare his opinion with yours. If you have back pains and are considering going to a chiropractor, you might want to know what your physician thinks of the idea. On the other hand, your primary care physician might recommend a therapy with which you would not be comfortable.

For instance, a friend once consulted an ear, nose, and throat doctor who had been highly recommended to her. After a short discussion of her overall health, the doctor advised her to try acupuncture. This was not something my friend wanted to do and she ultimately chose another physician.

If your opinions don't jibe with those of your health care professional, you should consider going elsewhere. The bottom line is that you must trust your doctor's recommendations. If you don't like and respect the doctor, and if your philosophy of health care is different from his, you'll probably resist any suggestions for treatment.

## THERE ARE SO MANY DIFFERENT KINDS OF DOCTORS OUT THERE. HOW DO I KNOW WHICH DOCTOR DEALS WITH WHICH PROBLEM?

This answer involves understanding the world of medicine. Picture this world as comparable to a video game. You start at level one and your goal is to get over some small hurdles and/or to combat a slow-moving enemy. As the game progresses, the hurdles become larger and the combatants more strenuous.

The world of medicine is built on the same principle. You start with first-level doctors, who get you past the smaller hurdles (most common illnesses, small accidents, cuts and abrasions) and help you to fight well-known enemies such as viruses and infections.

You overcome the various obstacles of your medical problems with this doctor until these hurdles become larger and the enemies get stronger, when you have to go on to second-level doctors. You continue to various levels (or specialists)—third, fourth, fifth—until you reach the level that has the doctor who can deal with your problem. Thus sometimes the appropriate doctor may be on the first level and sometimes he may be on the fifth.

## WHO ARE THE FIRST-LEVEL DOCTORS?

The first level is the family physician, also called the primary health care professional (a modern-day version of the old general practitioner). The family physician has been trained in all the specialties that make up the second level of the medical organization.

The primary health care professional is usually the one you consult first when you are having a problem. If the problem is diagnosed as serious (meaning that further attention is needed), the primary health care professional can act as a guide to the various levels of specialists.

## WHAT ARE THE SPECIALTIES THAT MAKE UP THE SECOND LEVEL?

The second-level specialties are: internal medicine, obstetrics and gynecology, pediatrics, psychiatry, and surgery.

## WHAT DOES EACH SPECIALTY DO?

*Internal medicine* is concerned with the diagnosis and treatment of all disease in people 18 years of age and older. It includes such fields as gastroenterology (the study of the digestive system), cardiology (the study of the heart and functions relating thereto), and endocrinology (the study of glands and hormones).

*Obstetrics* and *gynecology* make up the specialty concerned with any problems that relate to women specifically because they are women (after the onset of puberty).

*Pediatrics* deals with any problems relating to children from birth to age 18.

*Psychiatry* deals with mental, emotional, or behavioral disorders.

*Surgery* is the branch of medicine concerned with diseases and conditions that require an operation or something to be done that will physically modify the body's anatomy.

## WHAT ARE THE SPECIALTIES THAT MAKE UP THE THIRD LEVEL?

Each specialty has many subspecialties. For example, a subspecialty in pediatrics would be pediatric neurology or pediatric cardiology. There are subspecialists in internal medicine, such as the cardiologist (who deals with the heart), the gastroenterologist (who deals with digestive disorders), the neurologist (who deals with the nervous system), the rheumatologist (who deals with diseases of the body tissues such as muscles and joints), or the pulmonologist (who deals with diseases of the lungs). Subspecialties in surgery may involve the head and neck surgeon, the neurosurgeon (who deals with the nervous system), the orthopedist (a bone specialist), or the vascular surgeon (who deals with blood vessels). Within obstetrics and gynecology, one has subspecialists in terms of gynecologic oncologists (who test female cancers) or infertility specialists. In psychiatry, subspecialists may include child psychologists and specialists in addictive disorders or anxiety disorders.

## WHAT ARE THE SPECIALTIES THAT MAKE UP THE FOURTH LEVEL?

Subspecialties can be broken down even further, into sub-subspecialties. An example of this in pediatrics would be a neonatal cardiologist, a doctor who deals specifically with intensive care for newborns as it relates to ventilator control in respirators. A fourth-level doctor in surgery might be the neurosurgeon who specializes in pediatric neck surgery or the dermatologist who specializes in oncologic histopathology (the study of cancer cells). Another fourth-level doctor might be the psychiatrist who specializes in adult children of alcoholics as a subspecialty of the specialty in addictive disorders.

## SHOULD I GO TO A FAMILY PHYSICIAN FIRST OR CAN I GO DIRECTLY TO A SECOND-, THIRD-, OR FOURTH-LEVEL SPECIALIST?

It is usually a good idea to visit a primary care physician before you consult a specialist. The chest pains you are having, which you think are sure signs of heart disease, may turn out to be a digestive problem. Thus you may go to a cardiologist when you should really be seeing an internist. If you see a primary care physician first, he or she can probably tell you whether you do indeed have heart disease and refer you to the appropriate doctor.

Some women prefer to use their gynecologist as their primary (first-level) physician. And it's not unusual for parents to take children to their pediatricians for care that could be given by their family doctor.

In smaller communities, the lines between specialties often become blurred. In a town where there are no cardiologists, for example, the internal medicine physician is also the cardiologist. In a large city, it's not necessary for a family physician or an internist to practice cardiology when there is a cardiologist right down the hall.

## ARE THERE PHYSICIANS WHO DEAL SPECIFICALLY WITH THE OLDER MEMBERS OF THE POPULATION?

A recently established specialty is that of gerontology, which deals with the "geriatric population." This new specialty is comparable in some ways to the pediatric specialty, which has been in existence for a long time. The specialty of gerontology was developed because of the ever-increasing percentage of older people in the population, and as a result of the aging of the baby boomers and the advances in medical technology and public health care.

## WHAT IF I HAVE A PREFERENCE AS TO WHETHER I SEE A MALE OR A FEMALE DOCTOR?

Ideally, you should be looking for the best doctor you can find. But you should also feel comfortable and trust your doctor, so gender might be a deciding factor for you. If a doctor is listed as "Dr. Smith," you have no way of knowing whether that doctor is a man or a woman. Call the receptionist and ask. If you do have a preference, check it out before you waste a trip to the office.

## WHEN SHOULD I GO TO THE EMERGENCY ROOM?

To answer this question properly, you must first think temporally—that is, think in terms of how fast you need to see somebody. The question then becomes, "Is this so serious that I need to be seen immediately?"

Many physicians will deal with "minor" emergencies right in the office. For example, if you have a sore throat with intense pain, you need to see someone immediately. Usually, your regular doctor will fit you in for an emergency visit. (In Section 2, we discuss establishing emergency procedures with your physician.)

The emergency room was created to take care of extreme cases that need immediate attention. If you have had an accident, have broken a bone, or have a bad burn, a very deep cut, an excessively high fever, or any condition that seems life threatening, go to the emergency room.

Today, emergency room care is becoming an established specialty in the field of medicine. However, the emergency doctor isn't meant to take the place of your routine physician; she is usually someone you've never seen before and will probably never see again. She'll treat the problem to the point where it becomes stable and then make a referral to your primary health care physician or to an appropriate specialist.

## I'VE RECENTLY HEARD OF SOMETHING CALLED AN URGENT CARE CENTER. WHAT IS THAT?

The Urgent Care Centers are generally a cross between an emergency room and a doctor's office. They are set up to get you in and out quickly. They may be called by other names (such as Doctors' Care Center or Need Care Incorporated).

Like the emergency room, Urgent Care Centers are set up to take care of immediate problems, but they also take care of minor emergencies, such as a very sore throat or an infected cut. They are fast-service establishments, a little like the fast food chains, but they can be useful if your doctor is not available and you need fast treatment.

## WHEN SHOULD I GO TO AN URGENT CARE CENTER?

Most of the problems that are taken care of at the Urgent Care Center can also be taken care of by a primary health care professional. Thus these centers are generally attended by people who don't have primary care physicians.

If your usual doctor is unavailable and you feel you need immediate care, you might try an Urgent Care Center. Its drawback, like that of the emergency room, is that there is no continuity. You may see a different doctor every time you go there. However, no doctor-patient relationship is intended to be established; the centers are designed for one-time, isolated illnesses that do not require long-term care.

You should also be aware of the fact that most of these care centers don't accept insurance. That way, they cut down on paperwork and the extra personnel needed to handle it. Most centers require immediate payment at the time of the visit.

SECTION 2

# SMART QUESTIONS TO ASK WHEN CHOOSING A DOCTOR

Here's the setup: You've been promoted to a new job in a middle-size city in a state you have never even visited before. For the past two weeks, you have been experiencing minor stomach irritation and have decided that you need to see a doctor. Where do you go?

First you try the "Yellow Pages." There are many names listed, none of which mean anything to you. How do you choose? Should you start with Dr. Allan and go straight through to Dr. Zelig? This doesn't seem the answer. What next?

You don't know many people in this city, so you ask some co-workers for recommendations. You get three different names. The dilemma still remains—how do you choose?

Getting recommendations is probably the best way to

begin. It gives you somewhere to start and you can use the recommended doctor as a basis for comparison. But choosing a doctor is a very personal decision, and you should not base your choice solely on another person's opinion. The only way you can find out whether a doctor is right for you is by asking questions.

Some of the factors involved are personal; others are more practical in nature. For instance, asking the doctor questions about his degree or background, or how he feels about certain issues, will give you a good idea of how he thinks and of whether or not his philosophy agrees with yours. Other questions will give you factual information about office hours, the doctor's availability, and payment plans.

You may not choose to ask the doctor all 31 questions in this section. But you do want to ask enough questions to get the information you need. You also want to find out how willing this doctor is to answer any questions you might have, and how you react to the doctor's manner and attitudes.

You may choose to ask the staff some of these questions. You should be able to ask questions of anyone in the office, not just the doctor.

Everyone wants to feel safe and taken care of. If you're healthy, you want to know that your doctor takes an interest in your remaining that way. If you're sick, you want to know that you can go to someone you trust, someone who cares about you and who will do her best to make you better.

An unhappy patient is not a healthy patient. If you are unhappy with your medical care, it can affect the quality of your whole life. Choosing a doctor is a very important decision; if a doctor does not understand your need to ask questions, then perhaps you should find someone else.

A doctor-patient relationship is not based just on the doctor's giving advice and treatment and the patient following orders. A doctor-patient relationship is based on a mutual understanding, one that goes beyond purely medical matters and involves personality, politics, and philosophy, and a general understanding of each other as human beings.

## WHAT IS YOUR DEGREE?

These days, it seems that almost everyone gets to be called doctor. You want to know exactly the kind of doctor with whom you are dealing. A chiropractor's full title, for instance, is doctor of chiropractic; an osteopath (who uses a combination of chiropractic and traditional medicine) is a doctor of osteopathy. Some alternative care practitioners, such as alopaths or naturopaths, refer to themselves as doctors, although they may not have medical degrees. Sometimes we assume that they're doctors of medicine simply because they are in the healing profession.

There have even been cases where people have simply set themselves up as doctors. For example, in Redbird, Kentucky, a few years ago, a man who called himself Doc Randall prescribed drugs and practiced medicine for years before it was finally discovered that he had no medical degree whatsoever.

Although Doc Randall is certainly the exception to the rule, if you're looking for an M.D., make sure the person you're seeing is an M.D. Usually, the doctor's license is displayed prominently on the wall. If you have any questions, call your local Board of Medical Licensure.

## WHERE DID YOU DO YOUR TRAINING?

It's not necessary for a doctor to go to Harvard Medical School to be a good doctor, but the answer to this question can give you a better picture of this person and his history. Ask where the doctor went to school and where he did his residency. This will give the doctor an opportunity to discuss his background and afford you a chance to learn more about the doctor as a person. Knowing some of the personal details of his life can help you see the doctor as a "mere mortal," rather than as an intimidating authority figure.

You may feel that you would be better off with some-one who attended the "best" schools. However, the "best" schools don't always produce the best doctors, so you should not rely on this information alone when mak-ing your choice.

Some students go abroad to be trained. These are peo-ple who are extremely determined to be doctors and will go wherever they can obtain the necessary training. Often they have to learn another language, and learn it well enough to read complicated medical textbooks (which are difficult enough to read in English) in order to earn a med-ical degree. One has to respect people who are willing to go through all of that in pursuit of their goals.

## IN WHICH STATES ARE YOU LICENSED TO PRACTICE?

Since each state licenses doctors through its own board, a doctor has to apply to each state in which she wishes to practice for permission to do so.

Dr. Strauss relates: "When I did my residency in West Virginia, I had a license to practice there. When I decid-ed to start my practice in Kentucky, I applied for a license in that state. For a while, before I actually moved to Kentucky, I had licenses for both places and was able to practice in both West Virginia and Kentucky. Some doctors maintain licenses in more than one state; how-ever, the majority of doctors keep a license only for the state in which they currently practice."

The practical reason for asking this question has to do with prescriptions. Pharmacists are bound by state law to fill prescriptions by doctors who are licensed by the state in which the pharmacist is practicing. If you are in a New Jersey pharmacy and your doctor is licensed in Pennsylvania, she cannot call in a prescription for you unless she is also licensed in New Jersey.

## ARE YOU A BOARD-CERTIFIED SPECIALIST?

To be board certified, one must complete a residency training program and pass a national board examination, which must be retaken at intervals to retain board certification.

If a physician is board certified, you automatically know two things about him. One is that the person was rigorously trained and exposed to all areas of his specialty (for the family physician, this effectively means all areas of medicine), and the second is that he was willing to put up with at least two extra years of hard work and study in order to enhance his ability as a physician.

Many hospitals require that their affiliated specialists be board certified. There is no guarantee that a board-certified specialist is a better doctor than one is not board-certified. But asking a question like this can give you a good idea of the doctor's overall attitude toward answering your questions.

## WHAT DID YOU SCORE ON YOUR BOARD EXAM?

If you are really bold, you may want to ask this question to determine how much of the current medical vernacular your physician knows. A 90 percentile indicates an extraordinary grasp of the facts that fill the pages of the standard American medical texts and journals.

However, doctors who overvalue the accumulation of facts tend to relate to patients less as human beings. If you're lucky, you can get a physician who is able to do both—relate to you as a person and have a veritable wealth of medical knowledge.

## HOW DO YOU KEEP UP WITH THE LATEST DEVELOPMENTS IN YOUR FIELD?

Does this doctor read medical journals or go to educational seminars? If so, you might want to ask which ones, and perhaps peruse a copy or two of the journals. Much of the popular medical literature that physicians get today can be read and enjoyed by anyone with an interest in medicine. Your doctor might even be persuaded to lend you a copy of a publication he has already read.

Other questions you might ask in this area are: "What conferences have you recently attended?" "Do you participate in any continuing medical education?" "Do you do any writing?" "Do you do any teaching?"

## WHAT MEDICAL SOCIETIES OR ORGANIZATIONS DO YOU BELONG TO?

Once again, this question is designed to tell you something about the doctor's attitudes and personality. Is this someone who seeks out the company of others in her profession? Is she someone who values the feedback and ideas she may gain from colleagues? Is she an active participant in these organizations or does she just pay her membership dues and never attend meetings?

Her answers can also give you clues as to her concern

about the community. Medical associations, especially the local chapters, often act as springboards for community services. For instance, the Madison County Medical Association (of which Dr. Strauss is an active member) recently sponsored a health fair at which community residents could receive free blood pressure and cholesterol tests. You could ask the doctor, "Does your medical association sponsor any community activities? What is your participation in those activities?"

## WHAT ARE THE CURRENT HEALTH MAINTENANCE ISSUES OF WHICH I SHOULD BE AWARE?

A doctor should be willing to take the time to discuss issues of health maintenance, as well as the treatment of illnesses. For instance, a doctor who is interested in health maintenance may advise you to have a cholesterol count taken, even though you appear to be perfectly healthy. But he should also be willing to talk about all the different studies that have recently appeared regarding the questionable signficance of cholesterol levels in heart disease.

You could ask about the pros and cons of various exercise programs—jogging and aerobics, for example. You need to weigh the benefits of these activities for the heart and circulation systems against the possible damage to muscles and joints. If you're interested in being your own health advocate, your physician should be prepared to discuss health maintenance issues with you.

## WHERE CAN I GET MORE INFORMATION ABOUT THE ISSUES WE'VE BEEN DISCUSSING?

In the discussion of health maintenance, the physician should be able to refer you to sources of information that will allow you to study up on and formulate your own opinions concerning ways you can improve your health.

## MAY I SEE YOUR EXAMINING ROOMS?

A doctor's examining room may be very indicative of the way that he wants to treat his patients. I've heard that some pediatricians crawl around on their hands and knees when designing their offices so that they can see the rooms from a child's-eye view. A doctor who does that is bound to be a warm, caring person. If you're in the process of choosing a doctor, you probably want to take the office environment into account.

If you walk into the examining room and the thermostat is at 40 degrees and you can see icicles hanging from the faucets, ask why the temperature is kept at such a low level. You might find out it's because the doctor's secretary is going through menopause and has hot flashes, as is the case in Dr. Strauss's office. "Molly is very apologetic," he explains, "but says this is something she has to do, otherwise she wouldn't be able to function or think coherently. It's something I can live with, and my patients have been very understanding." If a situation like this is not acceptable to you, look for another doctor.

Take a look at the seats in the waiting room. Are they hard, wooden seats that you wouldn't feel comfortable sitting on for a few hours? Or are they deep, soft, luxurious seats that would be difficult for an older patient to get into and out of?

What about the exam tables? Are they modern or are they from back in the mid-1950s? Are you interested in a doctor who keeps an up-to-date stock of furniture and supplies or is this something that's not high on your list of priorities?

## DO YOU ALLOW SMOKING IN YOUR OFFICE?

If you have emphysema or a severe pulmonary problem, a nonsmoking office could be a deciding factor in choosing a doctor. Even if you don't have any such illness, you may want to choose a doctor whose attitudes toward smoking are the same as yours.

## I PREFER TO USE YOU AS MY FAMILY DOCTOR, BUT TO SEE MY GYNECOLOGIST AS WELL. DO YOU HAVE A PROBLEM WITH THAT?

It's important to know how your physician feels about this kind of arrangement. Some family physicians take pride in their ability to do specialty work and would prefer to do their own Pap smears, minor surgery, or internal-medicine workups in their office.

However, it's not at all unusual for families to maintain the family physician as the central unifying force for medical care, while using other specialists as the need arises.

## IS THIS A SOLO PRACTICE OR ARE YOU A PART OF A GROUP?

If it's a group practice, you want to know if you'll be seeing the same doctor every time. If you won't, you want to know how many doctors are in the group. If it's important to you to build a strong relationship with one doctor, a solo practice may be better for you.

## HOW LONG HAVE YOU BEEN PRACTICING IN THIS AREA?

It's comforting to know that a physician has been in an area for a long time and has many ties to the community.

This is an important issue for many people, according to Dr. Strauss. "I don't know how many times a patient has asked, 'How long have you been here, Doc?' The next question inevitably is, 'How long are you staying?' Patients don't want to get involved with a doctor, only to have him leave. In my part of the country, doctors come and go all the time. Patients are constantly lamenting to me about the fact that just when they thought they'd found a great doctor, he moved off. Patients get attached to doctors, and they don't like to make attachments if they think the doctor isn't going to stick around."

Statistically, doctors move a lot, but they move most often in the first few years of their practice. A doctor who has been in the area only a year or two is much more likely to move than someone who's been in the area for ten or twenty years.

## HOW CAN I CONTACT YOU IF AN EMERGENCY ARISES WHEN YOUR OFFICE IS CLOSED?

Some doctors are hard to contact in an emergency; some are impossible. Most doctors make sure that another doctor is available to handle emergencies if they cannot be reached. Are you satisfied with the arrangements this doctor has made? Is there a simple procedure for you to follow? Did the doctor explain it to you clearly? It's important that you understand the process before an actual emergency arises.

## HOW DO YOU FEEL ABOUT MY CONTACTING YOU AFTER OFFICE HOURS OR ON WEEKENDS?

Some doctors don't mind taking calls in off-hours and feel that it's just another part of medical practice. Others may say that they prefer their privacy to be respected and that there are other means of obtaining treatment in emergency situations.

You might ask your doctor if she minds you calling her at home if necessary. Some physicians will be glad to give you their number. And some doctors have a telephone at home that is connected to their office phone, so that they are automatically contacted if you call the office after hours.

You should also take into account the type of doctor involved. As a general rule, the more specialized the doctor, the less is the inclination to take after-hours calls. However, there are certain specialists who recognize the fact that emergencies will occur and that the primary care physicians will need to contact them, even if the patients are not able to. For instance, if you were having a heart attack, you would probably call your primary care physician, who would then contact your cardiologist, regardless of the time of day.

There are other specialties where one generally would not expect emergencies to arise. Such specialists will not encourage after-hour calls. For example, it's very rare to hear of a dermatologic emergency—although they do happen. My friend Monica is a model. One Saturday morning, Monica woke up with mysterious scaly patches on her face and arms—and she was scheduled to appear live in a televised fashion show that evening. She tried desperately to find her dermatologist, but could not. She eventually located an allergist who was able to help. "I make a living by my looks," Monica told me later. "The next day I called my dermatologist and got his after-hours number. You never know who you're going to need in an emergency!"

Your doctor's attitude may also depend on where you live. In a large metropolitan area where there are more after-hour facilities and emergency rooms or Urgent Care

Centers, the doctor may be less amenable to being called at home than in a small town where the emergency room facilities are limited.

## HOW MANY PATIENTS DO YOU BOOK EACH HOUR?

The answer to this question should give you some indication of how long the doctor will be able to spend with each patient. There are some physicians who purposely overbook—like the airlines do—so that if one person doesn't show up, there will be another to take that person's place.

If the doctor is booking ten patients an hour, that leaves approximately six minutes per visit. And that's assuming that the doctor doesn't have to take a four-minute phone call during your visit, leaving him two minutes to see you. If you prefer to spend more time with the doctor, go to someone who doesn't schedule as many patients in one hour.

## HOW LONG DO PATIENTS USUALLY HAVE TO WAIT BEFORE THEY ARE SEEN?

There's nothing more frustrating than arriving at a doctor's office on time for an appointment and having to wait more than three hours before you actually see the doctor.

Some doctors' offices, and many clinics, are run on a first-come, first-served basis. This is like lining up for tickets at Madison Square Garden hours or days before a game or a sell-out concert. It was worth the wait to get good seats. So if you really like the doctor, you may not mind the wait.

If you can, check with some of the doctor's current patients and find out how long they usually have to wait before they are seen.

## WHAT IS THE BEST TIME OF DAY TO MAKE AN APPOINT-MENT? WHEN IS THE OFFICE LEAST CROWDED?

Naturally, if doctors have evening and weekend hours, the office will be most crowded at these times. It is also likely to be jammed when it opens in the morning and near closing at night. Ask the receptionist when the office is least crowded, and if your schedule allows you to make your appointment then, you won't have to spend so much time in the waiting room.

## DO I NEED TO COME EARLY FOR MY APPOINTMENT?

Sometimes physicians' offices will give you an appointment and expect you to arrive 15 minutes early so that certain preparatory procedures can be carried out. Vital signs need to be taken, laboratory tests may need to be done, or forms may need to be filled out, especially if this is your first visit. A question like this can be asked over the telephone before you set out for the doctor's office.

## WITH WHAT HOSPITAL OR HOSPITALS ARE YOU AFFILIATED?

If you should require hospitalization, will you be happy with this doctor's affiliation? Check out the hospital's track record and reputation when you're not in a crisis situation—you won't want to spend the time when you're ill and anxious.

Ask around. Find out if any of your friends or co-workers have ever been to this hospital. You may want to visit the hospital yourself and see what your reaction is. (See Section 10 for questions pertaining to hospital procedures.)

## WHAT ARE YOUR FEES AND PAYMENT POLICIES?

Besides knowing how much the doctor charges, you want to know what kinds of insurance she will or will not accept, whether she will accept Medicare as payment in full, and whether the doctor's staff processes insurance claims or it is up to you to do so. You don't want to run into any surprises when you receive the bill.

## DO YOU ACCEPT ASSIGNMENT WITH MY INSURANCE POLICY?

Don't wait until after you've been examined to find out that the doctor you're seeing does not have an arrangement with your insurance company. This is a particularly important question with the new types of insurance organizations (such as health maintenance organizations—or HMOs as they are commonly known—and private pay organizations), which allow you to use only a select list of doctors.

Accepting assignment is the insurance company's way of indicating the relationship between the patient and the doctor. The insurance company has to ask the doctor, "Will you accept having this patient assigned to you?" If the doctor agrees, she also accepts the payment terms of the insurance company.

If the doctor accepts assignment, the insurance company will pay her directly. If the doctor doesn't accept assignment, the money sometimes goes directly to you as the patient and you are responsible for paying the doctor. Under most circumstances, HMO-type companies won't pay either you or the doctor if you go to someone who doesn't accept assignment.

## WHY DON'T YOU ACCEPT ASSIGNMENT?

If your doctor doesn't accept assignment, you want to find out the reasons for her decision. One reason could be that the doctor might not get as much from an insurance company as she would if she were to bill you privately. An insurance company may have a top dollar limit for a particular kind of doctor or treatment and will not pay beyond that limit.

Suppose you go to a dermatologist for an initial consultation and her fee for the visit is $100. Your insurance company, however, has an $80 limit on initial dermatologic consultations. So the doctor may decide that she will bill you directly for the full $100, while you get the $80 the insurance company will reimburse. Thus the visit will cost you $20 of your own money.

## WILL YOU ACCEPT THE INSURANCE PAYMENT OR WILL I HAVE TO PAY AS WELL?

Sometimes doctors will accept the insurance payment, but then expect you to make up the difference between what the insurance company pays them and the full amount of their bill. If the dermatologist above gets $80 from the insurance company, she may ask you to pay the additional $20. Some doctors will take the $80 from the insurance company and leave it at that.

## MUST I PAY YOU NOW OR CAN I WAIT TO BE REIMBURSED BY THE INSURANCE COMPANY?

A doctor may prefer that you pay the full amount at the time of the visit. In that way, the doctor is assured of receiving $100, while you have to wait for the insurance company to send the $80 it will pay for the visit.

Although it seems obvious that a doctor would prefer to be paid up front, it's possible that he will change his usual policy if you ask.

## WILL YOUR OFFICE HELP ME FILL OUT THE FORMS FOR THE INSURANCE COMPANY?

Some doctors' offices advise you to take the forms and fill them out yourself. Others fill out insurance forms as a service to the patient.

## IS THERE AN ADDED CHARGE FOR HELPING ME FILL OUT THE INSURANCE COMPANY FORMS?

Occasionally, a doctor's office will tack on a small helper's fee for filling out the forms. This is definitely something you should know beforehand.

## IF I DON'T HAVE INSURANCE, DO YOU EXPECT PAYMENT AT THE TIME OF THE VISIT OR CAN I PAY YOU WHEN I GET THE MONEY? CAN YOU BILL ME AND LET ME SEND YOU THE MONEY?

Some doctors the insist that full payment be made at the time of the visit. Others will allow you to arrange an installment payment plan.

Doctors can be very understanding when it comes to patients' bills. Dr. Strauss admits to having accepted eggs and nuts when patients had no other means of payment.

## WHO'S IN CHARGE OF YOUR COLLECTION?

Some doctors don't deal with the money aspects of their practice themselves. It's often difficult for a doctor who tries to be a caring and loving individual and an advocate for your health and well-being to be a money collector as well. Many doctors see these as conflicting roles. They distance themselves as much as possible from the money issue and hand over the collection of payment to other people within the practice, usually the financial manager of a large office or a nurse or secretary in a smaller office.

## WHAT IS YOUR POLICY CONCERNING MISSED APPOINT-MENTS?

We all know how busy doctors are, and there are doctors who do charge patients for missed appointments in order to discourage such behavior. Be sure you ask what the policy is. Some doctors will charge only if you miss without calling, others will charge if you call less than 24 hours in advance, and still others don't charge at all for missed appointments.

# SECTION 3

## SMART QUESTIONS TO ASK ABOUT TESTS AND EXAMINATIONS

Suppose you have a persistent cough that's been hanging on for two weeks and isn't getting any better. Or you're having stomach problems that are gradually getting worse. Or you simply don't feel well and you can't explain why. What do you do? You make an appointment and go in to see the doctor.

The first thing that happens is that the doctor asks you a series of questions. It's important that you answer these questions to the best of your ability because they give the doctor vital clues about your physical past, present, and future.

But it's also important that you ask the doctor such questions as, "Why are you asking me this?" "Why are you interested in my family history?" "What are you looking for?" "What does my past medical history have to do with this?" "What do allergies have to do with this?"

Has this ever happened to you? You go to the doctor with a headache and she asks if anyone else in your family has headaches. Her reaction to your answer is a shake of the head and a low "Hmmmmm." Her reaction makes you so nervous that you assume there's something seriously wrong—and you don't say another word.

The next time this happens, don't get nervous—ask questions. Ask her, "Why did you react that way?" "What was the significance of asking that question?" "What was the significance of my answer?" "How does it affect what you're thinking?"

The next thing that is likely to happen is that the doctor will conduct a preliminary examination in her office. Once again, ask questions all along the way. Find out exactly what it is that the doctor is doing and what she's looking for.

Your job is to ask, "How's my blood pressure doing?" "How's my pulse?" "How's my respiration?" "How's my temperature?" You want to know why the doctor is interested in these bodily functions, what they are, and how you're doing.

The doctor may recommend that you undergo further testing. There are three basic reasons why a doctor might suggest that a particular test or exploratory procedure be done:

- She has a pretty good idea of what your problem is, but wants to be absolutely sure.
- Your symptoms could be indicative of several different things and testing would narrow down the possibilities.
- The doctor is unable to make a diagnosis and needs more information.

If your doctor suggests further tests or examinations, you want to know which of the three categories they fall into. Ask, "Why do I need these tests? Is it because you think you know what's wrong or because you don't know what the problem is?"

Questions should be asked whether you're having your blood pressure taken in the doctor's office or are preparing for a complex hospital procedure. This section includes the questions you may want to ask when any tests or examinations are recommended or performed. Once again, you need not ask every question provided in this section. A doctor may not have time to go into detailed explanations of every routine procedure. But she should be willing to give you a brief idea of what she's doing and why's she's doing it.

You are not asking the doctor to make a diagnosis before she has all the facts. But it's important that you understand the why, what, when, and how of anything that affects your body. A clear understanding of the testing procedures will let you know that these tests are being done *for* you, not *to* you.

Asking questions also alleviates some of the fear and anxiety that often accompanies these procedures. It's not what we know that scares us; it's what we don't know. You make the unknown the known by asking questions.

Finally, asking questions forces the doctor to relate to you and lets her know that you expect to be involved in your health care. Asking questions also lets her know that you want the best care you can possibly get. Make the doctor think: think about what she's doing; think about what she's going to do; think about how she can best serve you.

## WHAT IS THE NAME OF THE TEST THAT'S BEING DONE AND HOW IS IT SPELLED?

When your doctor recommends a specific test or procedure, write down the name immediately. You may want to discuss the recommendation with another doctor, with your family, or with the lab technician. These tests often have complicated names and spellings, so having the test name written down in front of you will make it much easier for you to refer to it.

## WHY ARE YOU DOING THIS PARTICULAR EXAMINATION? WHAT ARE YOU LOOKING FOR?

Being a doctor is very much like being a detective. The doctor starts with general information (perhaps even as general as, "I don't feel well") and then begins to search for clues to tell him what's wrong. Tests and examinations give him the clues he needs to solve the crime or, in this case, to diagnose the illness.

Dr. Strauss gives this example: "A complaint that I (and most other doctors) hear over and over again is, 'Doctor, I'm so tired all the time.' Usually, making a diagnosis in a case like this means real detective work. Fatigue is a difficult issue, because there can be a great variety of causes.

"I'd start by giving you a thorough physical exam, and asking questions regarding your physical health. I'd find out if there are any other symptoms besides lack of energy.

"If I still can't find an answer, my next step would involve chemical tests, such as blood, renal (kidney), and thyroid tests. If all these are negative, I'd check out the psychological factors: How much sleep are you getting? How much work are you doing? What kind of stress are you under?

Asking the doctor questions as he examines you can help this process. If you know what he's looking for, you may be able to elaborate on what's bothering you or lead him to look in other directions. You want him to have as much information as possible so that he can make clear, logical deductions about what is wrong with you and how to fix it.

Also, asking these questions makes the doctor focus on what he is doing. You take away the sense that it is merely routine and make it into something new and exciting. Dr. Strauss adds, "Occasionally, you'll find doctors who feel they don't have time to discuss in detail why a test has been suggested. These doctors may decide to have the nurse talk to you about why the tests are being done. If that's acceptable to you, that's fine. My personal feeling is that, if I'm going to be taking a test, I want to know why. I don't want anybody to rush through anything where my health is concerned—or the health of my patients."

You need to ask these questions so that you learn the answer, so that the doctor thinks more clearly about the answer himself, and so that there develops between the two of you a feeling of participation in trying to solve the problem.

## WOULD YOU DESCRIBE IN DETAIL THE PROCEDURE YOU WANT ME TO UNDERGO?

Many tests and diagnostic procedures are relatively easy and not at all painful or frightening. Why spend time and sleepless nights worrying about a procedure that will take 15 minutes and an office visit? Having your blood pressure taken, for example, is a simple, painless test that's given all the time.

On the other hand, there are some procedures for which you should be prepared. They may even be painful. One such test would be an electromyogram (EMG). In an EMG, needles are stuck into a muscle to act as electrodes and measure electric currents. The results usually indicate a dysfunctional nerve and tell you why you're having weakness in that muscle. The test itself can be rather painful. You should know this beforehand so that you can mentally "psyche yourself up" for it.

## HOW DO I ARRANGE FOR THE LABORATORY TESTS YOU WANT DONE?

Most of the time, laboratories need specific information from the doctor. For one thing, the laboratory needs to know that the doctor has indeed ordered the test for the patient; if the lab doesn't receive the order, the lab work cannot be done. Patients have arrived at a lab only to find that no orders have been received and the test cannot be done.

Ask your doctor if she will be calling ahead to schedule the lab work for you or if you need to make the call, and whether or not you need to bring any specific orders with you.

## WHERE DO I GO FOR THESE TESTS?

Your doctor may have a special arrangement with a lab on the other side of town, but that doesn't mean you *have* to go to that lab. Find out what your options are.

## ARE THERE ANY SPECIAL PREPARATIONS FOR THESE TESTS?

Is there anything special you should or should not do before you take this test? You could waste a lot of time if you show up for your tests and find out then that you should not have eaten the night before. Don't assume that just because the doctor didn't say anything, you don't need to do anything. Better to ask than appear for the test, be turned away, and have to reschedule it.

Ask for details. If the doctor says, "Don't eat the night before the test," ask if she means that you should stop eating at 8:00 p.m. or at midnight. When you prepare for your test might make a difference, as well as how you prepare.

I learned this from personal experience. Several years ago,

before I learned to ask questions, I was scheduled to have a sonogram to check out a possible ovarian cyst. For that test, you're required to have a full bladder, which means you are asked to drink lots of fluids. I was told to drink eight glasses of water before the test. Being a dutiful patient, I did just that before I left the house. I then proceeded to board a bus to go to the doctor's office. Usually, I don't mind New York's traffic problems, but that day the city seemed particularly crowded and I was caught on the bus for more than 45 minutes. Discomfort is a polite word for my agony. Imagine how silly I felt when I got to the doctor's office and noticed several other patients drinking their glasses of water right there in the waiting room! If only I'd asked the doctor for advice on how best to prepare for this test.

## IS THERE A PARTICULAR TIME OF THE DAY TO HAVE THIS TEST DONE?

There are some tests that require you to be in the laboratory at certain times of the day. For example, blood sugar levels usually need to be tested first thing in the morning so that the test follows several hours of not eating. People scheduled for these tests are usually advised not to eat after dinner and also not to eat breakfast (except for water or coffee without sugar).

## DO I NEED TO DRESS ANY PARTICULAR WAY TO TAKE THIS TEST?

If you're taking a test like the cardiac exercise stress test, it's usually recommended that you come in your jogging clothes or something else that's loose and comfortable. You wouldn't want to show up in a dress or suit and be unable to take the scheduled test. It's better to ask and be sure.

## I MIGHT BE PREGNANT. DOES THAT MAKE A DIFFERENCE?

If you even suspect that you might be pregnant, this is a *question that must be asked.* It seems so obvious that it frequently gets missed, and it may be extremely important. Women who are pregnant are best not x-rayed, for example, except in emergencies—and then only with protection for their ovaries and the unborn child.

## DO YOU NEED TO KNOW IF I'VE EVER HAD THIS TEST DONE BEFORE?

Doctors frequently use previous tests for comparison with present measurements or levels. For example, if you've had an electrocardiogram (a measurement of electrical charges occurring during the heartbeat), the doctor will want to compare the new electrocardiogram with a previous one in order to determine whether or not any new cardiac damage has taken place.

## HOW WILL I FEEL DURING THE PROCEDURE? AFTER THE PROCEDURE IS OVER?

Some test procedures can be uncomfortable or even painful. It's best to find out what you're getting into so that you won't be taken by surprise if you start to feel queasy or experience pain.

Dr. Strauss adds that during certain procedures, a dye may be injected that can make you feel dizzy and lightheaded. If you don't know that this is a usual reaction, you may start to panic. He says, "I've known patients who have begun to feel strange and assume that the worst is happening, that they are dying. They become hysterical and demand that the procedure be stopped.

All this can be avoided by asking a few simple questions beforehand."

## ARE THERE ANY RISKS INVOLVED WITH THESE TESTS OR LABORATORY PROCEDURES?

This is a subject that is worth checking out. The fact is that there are risks involved with everything. Some of the risks the procedures pose may be rather obscure. "For example," says Dr. Strauss, "you may not know that one is cautioned against having an electrocardiogram during an electrical storm. I didn't learn this in medical school or in my residency and, in fact, was not aware of it until I got my first electrocardiograph and read the owner's manual.

"Other risks are more obvious. If you are in any way allergic to iodine or any of the components of the dyes sometimes used in x-rays, you could have a severe, or even fatal, reaction. In the rare case that your doctor has forgotten to ask you about any allergies, this question could save your life.

"There are also misconceptions about the risks of some tests. Many people think that there is a risk of contracting AIDS during a blood test. However, the needles now used in blood testing are sterile needles that are used once and thrown away. Although it is true that you can contract AIDS from shared needles, blood-test needles are disposed of after only one use. As with any other tests, if you have a question, ask it."

## ARE THERE ANY ADVERSE REACTIONS ASSOCIATED WITH THESE TESTS?

Adverse reactions are distinguished from risks in that an adverse reaction does not produce serious injury, although it might make you feel uncomfortable. For example, some people experience a sense of uncomfortable flushing during the injection of x-ray dyes.

Another adverse reaction that some people have is a feeling of claustrophobia during a CT scan, which requires that you stay perfectly still in an enclosed machine. I had a CT scan a few years ago, and no one warned me that this might happen. It was an extremely frightening experience. If I had been told what the procedure entailed and how I might react, I would have been able to prepare myself psychologically.

## AM I GOING TO BE SEDATED FOR THIS PROCEDURE?

There are some procedures that can be rather uncomfortable. If you're having colon problems, a doctor might suggest a colonoscopy. In this procedure, a tube is maneuvered through the descending colon, the transverse colon, and the ascending colon. Some doctors suggest that you be sedated so that you will be relaxed. Others believe that a colonoscopy is best done while you're awake and alert.

If the idea of being awake during this procedure scares you, you might want to get a second opinion about it, or perhaps find a doctor who will sedate you for the test.

## CAN THIS TEST BE DONE ON AN OUTPATIENT BASIS?

For some procedures, the doctor will want to admit you to the hospital and keep you there for a day or two. Other procedures can be undergone strictly as an outpatient—you come into the hospital or the doctor's office, you spend a few hours there and you leave.

When I had my lumpectomy done, one surgeon told me

he could remove the small tumor right in his office. This was comforting to hear because it made the whole procedure seem less threatening. I chose to have it done in the hospital, but I was glad to have the second option.

## HOW DO I FIND OUT THE RESULTS OF THESE TESTS?

Never assume that the doctor will contact you. Even if it is her policy to contact the patient, lab results can get lost—and a year later your abnormal Pap smear is found somewhere at the back of a drawer. You can become angry and annoyed with the physician for not having called you, but that's small comfort if you're now receiving chemotherapy for a malignancy that was missed because of lost test results.

"I know of a specific example," says Dr. Strauss, "in which a mammogram showed a questionable mass. However, the report was never returned to the doctor's office and the doctor did not follow up with the lab. Needless to say, the patient was quite upset when, a year later, she was diagnosed with breast cancer.

"It's true that the doctor never followed up. Doctors are human, and they get busy or simply forget. Had this patient called the office and requested her lab results, the doctor would have realized that the report had not been received."

If the doctor says she'll call you, find out when she plans to call. If you don't hear from her at that time, call the office and remind her that the test results are due.

## SHOULD I CALL YOUR OFFICE AT A SPECIFIC TIME TO GET MY RESULTS?

Most doctors have certain times when they are more easily reached. Often, when you call the doctor's office, you are asked to leave a message and told that the doctor will get back to you. Many doctors set aside certain times of the day specifically for returning telephone calls. Some will actually do this during their lunch hour, but most wait until after they have finished seeing patients for the day and spend this time returning calls from patients.

If you're asked to leave a message, find out an approximate time when the doctor will be calling you so that you don't wait by the phone all day, only to have the doctor make his return call during the one half-hour period you stepped out to pick up the kids.

## WHEN I CALL YOUR OFFICE, WHO WILL TELL ME THE TEST RESULTS?

Do you need to talk to the doctor herself or can you speak to the nurse or receptionist? Usually, the more complex the test, the more likely it is that you'll want to speak to the doctor personally. If you ask this question beforehand, you'll know that you have the right to insist on speaking to the doctor if the need should arise.

## WOULD YOU PLEASE EXPLAIN THE TEST RESULTS IN PLAIN ENGLISH SO THAT I CAN UNDERSTAND WHAT YOU'RE TALKING ABOUT?

Have you ever had this experience? Your doctor attempts to explain the results of the tests that you have taken and what the implications are for your future. You are listening intently, but it does not appear—except for a few words here and there—that the doctor is speaking English.

Dr. Strauss explains this phenomenon: "When I start

talking to patients, I really don't mean to talk over their heads. Unfortunately, occasionally I do.

"There are really two reasons for this. One is that I don't want to treat patients as if they are ignorant. I want to talk on the patient's level. Usually, I start by assuming that the patient knows a little more than he really does. I count on the patient's letting me know if I'm not being clear.

"There's another reason why doctors aren't always clear. When we talk to our nurses and colleagues, we frequently speak in medical jargon. Sometimes we forget that not everybody else knows the same jargon. So if you don't stop me when I start talking this way, I'll go on, not realizing I'm speaking a foreign language.

"Don't be afraid to ask questions when you don't know something. When you hear something that doesn't register, say, 'Stop. Wait a second. What does that mean?' And if you're afraid to ask what it means, then you should ask yourself, 'Why am I afraid to ask? What does *that* mean?'

"Doctors need to know when you don't understand what's going on. If you don't want to ask questions because you're embarrassed to look stupid in front of the doctor, you're only hurting yourself and your potential for improving your health. The only way you learn is by asking questions. I wouldn't go to a doctor who thinks I'm stupid because I ask questions."

## CAN I HAVE A COPY OF MY LAB RESULTS?

You might want to keep test results in your personal file. You can then refer to them if you switch doctors or if you go to a consulting doctor.

Another reason to keep your test results on file is if your problem is one that runs in your family. Such data could be very helpful in diagnosing or treating other family members.

## IS THIS TEST GOING TO TELL US SOMETHING SPECIFIC OR IS IT GOING TO TELL US SOMETHING GENERAL?

If it doesn't tell us something specific, what's the next step? Will I need more tests?

## WHAT IS CONSIDERED NORMAL FOR THESE TEST RESULTS?

You want to know what your test results are as compared with what the results would be for an average healthy person.

If you look at the actual test results that come back from the lab, chances are that you won't understand what you're seeing. The results will most likely appear as a set of numbers that mean nothing to you. That's why you must ask the doctor to explain exactly what all these numbers mean.

## IF THE RESULT IS NOT NORMAL, HOW ABNORMAL IS IT?

You can't judge test results by numbers alone. A blood count that is slightly elevated in one person, given the person's background, history, and present physical state, can mean that everything is in relatively good condition. In another person, the same elevated blood count could be cause for concern.

## WHAT DOES IT MEAN IF THE TESTS ARE VERY ABNORMAL?

Does it mean I'm fatally ill? According to Dr. Strauss, "Sometimes really abnormal tests don't tell us very much and sometimes they tell us a whole lot. For example, if you have an elevated erythrocyte sedimentation rate, it could mean just about anything. It could mean that you've got some sort of arthritic problem. It could mean that you've got some cancer somewhere. It could mean that you've got a generalized infection. It could mean a lot of things. In this case, an abnormal result doesn't tell us anything specific; it only means that something's wrong in a general way.

"There are other tests that tell you something very specific if they're abnormal. For example, a large white spot on a chest x-ray will indicate a definite problem in a very specific area of the body."

## HOW MUCH ARE THESE TESTS GOING TO COST?

If you have got limited resources, you should know that some of these tests can deplete your bank account. although some are relatively inexpensive, ranging from $5 to $15, other tests can run into hundreds of dollars. A CT scan is very expensive, for example, and that's not including the cost of the radiologist who will read the reports.

## WHOM DO I PAY TO HAVE THESE TESTS DONE?

Ask the doctor about the payment policy for the test or lab work. Some laboratories require payment at the time of the test and some will bill you. If your insurance will cover the test, you will need to have the correct forms and know how to fill them out.

# SECTION 4

## SMART QUESTIONS TO ASK WHEN A DIAGNOSIS HAS BEEN MADE

Your tests have been carried out and the results have come back positive. There is something wrong with you. What do you need to know?

This is a difficult time for you as a patient. You want to know what's wrong and you want to know what you should do about it, but you're frightened and you're not feeling well. It's hard to concentrate, and you'd rather not think about it at all. But you must think about it. You have a much better chance of a full recovery if you know what's wrong with you, what to expect, and what you can do to speed up the recovery process.

Years ago, it was a common philosophy among physicians that there was no need to tell the patient the details of an illness. Today, most doctors feel that it is your right to know what's going on inside your body.

However, it's up to you to let your doctor know that you want to be an active participant in fighting this illness. You need to keep asking questions until you're satisfied that you have all the answers.

Use this section as a guideline. Take the book with you to the doctor's office or write the questions down so that you won't forget to ask. And write down the doctor's answers so that you'll remember them later.

How does it help you to know exactly what's wrong with you? Often, you begin to feel better simply by gaining a clear understanding of what it is that's causing you stress, pain, and discomfort. All of these things can be exacerbated by fear and anxiety. If you can reduce your anxiety, you can lessen your pain and discomfort.

When you have a clear understanding of your illness, you also have a better understanding of the treatment. According to Dr. Strauss, "I've had many patients who have the attitude, 'I don't want to know what's wrong with me.' They don't ask me any questions, and I'm never sure whether or not they understand what I'm telling them. They actively avoid understanding the nature of their problem. In doing so, they actively avoid the treatment as well.

"An example of this is patient X, who has functional bowel disease. In this particular patient's case, it means that certain foods tend to cause severe cramping and alternating diarrhea and constipation. When this patient comes to the office, all she can think of is the fact that she's in pain. Any attempt to explain why the pain occurs is met with resistance. Therefore, any appropriate treatment that is recommended is also met with resistance. The treatment is, of course, to avoid those foods that tend to aggravate the bowels.

"Now, this patient doesn't want to hear that she's to be restricted from eating certain foods. She just wants to hear that the pain's going to go away, that somehow she's going to be made miraculously better."

Unfortunately, you can't depend on being made "miraculously better." But you can depend on questions to help you to:

- Get the information you need.
- Form a partnership between yourself and your doctor.
- Feel more in control of your own health and well-being.

## WHAT IS REALLY WRONG WITH ME?

After all has been said and done, this is perhaps the smartest question that you can possibly ask your physician. The question seems obvious, but it's surprising how many people actually fail to get a clear understanding of their problem.

The physician must take part of the responsibility for making sure that you know and understand the diagnosis. But if anything isn't clear or doesn't make sense to you, ASK THIS QUESTION until you understand the answer. You can't take care of yourself properly and effectively unless you know what the problem actually is.

## IS IT POSSIBLE FOR ME TO GO HOME AND TALK TO SOME OTHER PEOPLE BEFORE WE CONTINUE THIS CONVERSATION?

Suppose you're diagnosed with a serious illness, such as cancer. What's the first thing that happens? Usually, your mind goes blank. Mine certainly did. Nine years ago, when I heard the verdict, "Your tumor was malignant," I couldn't concentrate on anything for 24 hours.

You are in shock and nothing the doctor says is registering. You are no longer listening to her; you're thinking about what's going to happen to you. It's important to let the doctor know that you're not able to concentrate on what she's saying. You may want to bring someone else back to the office with you—someone who is able to remain calm and really hear and understand what is being said.

## WHAT IS THE CURE FOR THIS PROBLEM?

As stated earlier, there are very few miracle cures in medicine. Most cures take time and work and lots of energy. A cure may involve strict dietary limitations; it could require rigorous exercise or physical therapy. A cure may necessitate surgery, or it may mean a total change of life-style.

Sometimes patients are resistant to being cured. For example, people who are very overweight and have symptoms of heart disease often find it difficult to reduce their intake of fats and sweets to lose weight. Some people continue to smoke even after they've been diagnosed with lung cancer.

When my father was 60 years old, he had a heart attack. A neighbor, around the same age, had a heart attack one week later. Both men were warned to change their behavior.

My father lost 25 pounds and taught himself new ways of dealing with stress and anxiety. Our neighbor continued to drink, smoke, and eat lots of fatty foods. He died within a year. My father lived to be 78 years old.

In extreme cases, there may not be a cure for your particular problem. But there is almost always a course of action that can be taken to stave off the illness for as long as possible. Whatever your diagnosis, you should be aware of all your options for care and treatment. There will be more questions on this subject in the next section.

## IS THIS CONDITION GOING TO BE PERMANENT? IS IT SOMETHING I'M GOING TO HAVE ALL MY LIFE?

Some conditions are called chronic and some are called acute. A chronic condition is one that lasts for a long time. An acute condition is one that arises suddenly and doesn't last very long. Diabetes, for example, is a chronic condition, one that remains with you all of your life (I use diabetes often as an example because it is such a common disease—most people have at least a basic idea of what it is).

Says Dr. Strauss, "It's possible to control some chronic conditions through diet or medication, but it's not always possible to cure them. Patients who have been treated for high blood pressure for years and years may come to me and say, 'Look, Doc, I'm better now. I no longer have high blood pressure.' So we check the blood pressure and they're right—the pressure's pretty normal. They stop taking their medication.

"Then they say, 'My blood pressure is normal. Does this mean that I've been cured?' My response is that high blood pressure is something that you have all your life. If you're doing better now, it's not because the condition is gone, it's because you have been able to get it under control through diet or exercise."

## IF THIS IS A CHRONIC CONDITION, HOW WILL MY LIFE BE AFFECTED BY IT?

If you have a condition that will be with you for the rest of your life, you'll have to take care of it for the rest of your life. For instance, if you have diabetes, you may have to give yourself injections of insulin every day or remain on a special diet. Certain skin conditions are affected by light. If you have such a condition, you need to know that you can't be exposed to the sun for long periods, and that you should always carry sunscreen around with you and make sure that you wear wide-brimmed hats, and clothes that cover the skin while in the sun.

A chronic condition may not affect another person's life in the same way that it affects yours. If you've been a surfer for most of your life and you suddenly develop a chronic skin condition, it could require a major change in life-style. But if you're a computer operator and spend most of your time indoors anyway, the condition may not affect your life much at all.

## IS THIS A CONDITION THAT WILL BE WITH ME CONSTANTLY OR WILL IT RECUR INTERMITTENTLY?

There are certain conditions that are always with you. One example, according to Dr. Strauss, is hyperthyroidism, where the thyroid is not functioning properly. In that case, you will always need replacement thyroid hormones. Your energy and metabolism are dependent on this hormone; without it, you have feelings of fatigue and all of your systems slow down to the point where life becomes extremely unpleasant. The only way to remedy this situation is to take synthetic thyroid hormones, which will allow your body to function on a sustained normal level. This is a condition that is constant and will not change.

There are other types of conditions that come and go. Some people have migraine headaches, for instance. That doesn't mean they are plagued by migraines all the time. They may go for months, even years, without having any headaches. Then, because of an increase in stress or anxiety, or sometimes without any apparent reason, they may start having migraines weekly or daily.

## HOW OFTEN CAN I EXPECT THIS CONDITION TO RECUR?

This depends on the condition. Some arise cyclically on a regular basis, the way that pre-menstrual syndrome occurs regularly before menstruation. Others, such as allergies, for example, are seasonal and depend on the amount of pollen or ragweed in the air.

On the other hand, certain diseases or conditions recur without any apparent pattern. For instance, some types of leukemia may be in remission for years and then suddenly reappear for no discernible reason.

Chronic conditions are often affected by how well we treat ourselves. It's possible that as long as you relax, eat the right foods, get enough sleep, and take the prescribed exercise, you can remain healthy and forestall any recurrences of your illness. Such is the case with cardiovascular disease, which, with proper exercise, diet and life-style stress changes, can often be reversed. This contrasts sharply with a condition such as Alzheimer's disease, for which there is as yet no known cure or way to reverse the process.

## ARE THERE PARTICULAR SUBSTANCES OR SITUATIONS THAT WILL CAUSE A RECURRENCE?

You want to know if there are any foods, fabrics, plants, or stressful situations that can cause your condition to recur or to get worse.

Asthma, for example, is highly susceptible to outside influences. Certain types of allergens, molds, mildews, or even stress can exacerbate asthma. "I had a patient who would come to the office every time there was a family quarrel," says Dr. Strauss. "She lived with her husband and his parents, and she would come in whenever they had an argument. When she asked me what she could do to prevent her asthma from recurring, my response was, 'Move out.' When she finally did move out, her attacks ended."

## IS THIS DISEASE CONTAGIOUS?

A contagious disease is one that is spread by passing the causative agent of the disease (such as a bacterium or a virus) from one person to another. This is an important question to ask because you want to avoid spreading the disease whenever possible. You also want to know if you should be prepared for other members of your family coming down with the disease.

## IF THIS DISEASE IS CONTAGIOUS, EXACTLY HOW IS IT SPREAD?

Most childhood diseases are very contagious because the infections are airborne. When we are breathing in and out, we are taking moisture in and we are pushing moisture out. Bacteria live in these moisture droplets, and everyone around you will breathe them in as well. In fact, most childhood infections are so widespread because of the close contact in such areas as day-care centers, schools, and playgrounds—places where kids come into contact with large numbers of other children.

Contact is another means of spreading disease. Typhoid Mary fits into this category. She did her damage because infected bacteria would get into the food everywhere she went.

Other diseases are sexually transmitted. Given the rise of sexually transmitted diseases all over the country, it is urgent that you know whether your condition is contagious, and if it is, exactly how you can prevent anyone else from catching it.

## JUST HOW CONTAGIOUS IS THIS DISEASE?

You want to ask this question so that you know exactly what precautions you can take, if any, to keep the disease from spreading to anyone else. Some of the airborne contagions are impossible to avoid except by absolute isolation from anyone breathing. With other diseases that are contagious, you have to have intimate contact for long periods before they spread. You need to know which category your illness fits into and what you should be doing to avoid passing it on.

If you have measles, for example, you need to be very careful of even casual contact with other people. Measles is an airborne, highly contagious disease. AIDS, on the other hand, is not airborne, so casual contact with others will not spread the disease.

## WHAT STAGE OF CONTAGION AM I IN?

Some diseases are extremely contagious in their beginning stages, but are not contagious as they progress. Therefore, it's possible for you to spread a disease before you even know you have it.

For instance, you may be sneezing and coughing for three or four days and assume you have a cold. You go to work or to a meeting and don't give it a second thought. By the fourth day, however, little red dots begin to appear all over your body. You have chicken pox! Unfortunately, the most contagious period was the three or four days of sneezing and coughing, before the telltale symptoms appeared.

## IS THIS DISEASE GENETIC? DOES IT RUN IN MY FAMILY?

Your height, your body shape, and many other personal characteristics, including the color of your eyes, your hair and your skin, are determined by the genes you inherited from your parents or grandparents. There are many diseases that are handed down in the same way.

## IF THIS IS A GENETIC DISEASE, DOES THAT MEAN I'LL DEFINITELY GET IT OR THAT MY CHILDREN WILL DEFINITELY GET IT?

There are very few definites in life. If you are genetically predisposed to (or carry the genes for) a disease, you may or may not get it.

Diabetes is a good example once again. The fact that one of your parents, or even both of them, has diabetes does not automatically mean that you will have diabetes too. It probably means you have a predisposition toward getting it and will need to have regular tests and checkups to make sure you're healthy.

Another example concerns allergies. It's been well observed (although not absolutely proved) that parents with allergies tend to have children with allergies. Even within families, however, one child can develop severe allergies while a sibling never shows any signs at all. Both children may have the same predisposition, but only one ends up with the disease.

## IF I DO HAVE THIS GENETIC PREDISPOSITION, WILL I DEVELOP THE CONDITION TO THE SAME DEGREE THAT MY PARENT HAS IT?

There is a medical term known as penetrance, which means that genetic predisposition may not completely manifest in your body. Take something as common as baldness.

Your family may have the genes for baldness. Perhaps your father is completely bald and has been so since he was 20 years old. Will you be the same? Not necessarily. You may be only slightly bald at the age of 40 because the genes for baldness have not penetrated deep into your physical makeup.

## IF I HAVE THIS GENETIC PREDISPOSITION, SHOULD I HAVE CHILDREN?

Whether or not you have allergies or your father was bald at 20 most likely will not affect your decision to have children. But if you are a person with a genetic predisposition toward a more serious illness, this could be a major consideration in terms of family planning.

## IF THERE IS A GENETIC PREDISPOSITION, IS THERE ANYTHING I CAN DO TO PREVENT THE CONDITION FROM OCCURING IN ME OR IN MY CHILDREN?

This is a very important question to ask. For instance, if you have a predisposition to diabetes, it would be prudent for you to watch your diet and weight and get enough exercise. To do so may prevent you from developing the illness.

Allergies are another example. If you are allergic, or were allergic as a child, you should probably take precautions by desensitizing your home. That is, you should try to avoid potential allergens such as cats, dogs, pollens, or molds and mildews.

You can't prevent your child from having a predisposition to allergies, but by taking these precautions, you may prevent your child from developing problems.

## IS IT POSSIBLE THAT MY CONDITION IS NOT HEREDITARY, BUT IS CAUSED BY ENVIRONMENTAL FACTORS?

Heredity versus environment has been a controversial issue in science for a long time. Certain cancers, for instance, seem to be hereditary—but only appear if certain environmental factors are also present.

Every day we hear new reports of substances that are toxic or bad for our health. You can't avoid all of them every day of your life or you won't be able to live, work, and enjoy your family. Even sunshine can cause cancer, so there is no way to avoid all environmental influences. However, the more aware you are of the foods you eat, the water you drink, and the earth beneath your feet, the better are your chances of living a long and healthy life.

## WHAT ARE THE POSSIBLE COMPLICATIONS OF THIS DISEASE OR CONDITION?

This question could be a life-saver. If you are prepared for possible complications, you may be able to prevent them from occurring or to deal with them quickly and effectively if they do occur.

Suppose you've been diagnosed with juvenile-onset diabetes (a serious form of diabetes that appears in children and young adults). If you don't watch your blood sugar carefully and don't take your insulin precisely as instructed, you can expect any of a number of complications. It's important to know what these complications are. On the other hand, if you take too much insulin and your blood sugar drops too far, you'll become hypoglycemic and a different set of complications will arise.

Complications may evolve even if you have done

everything you've been advised to do, but if you're aware of the possibilities, you'll be better able to cope with the situation.

## WHAT ARE THE SYMPTOMS OF THESE COMPLICATIONS?

To stay with the diabetes example, it's possible that you may not realize you've taken either too much or too little insulin. Therefore, it's important to know the signs and signals that mean that something is wrong. If your blood sugar has gone up too high, you'll experience symptoms like fatigue and nausea. If you get a bad headache, start shaking, and feel extremely light-headed, your blood sugar is probably too low. If you are prepared for the possibility of these complications, you can get specific instructions as to what to do if they should appear.

## ARE YOU POSITIVE THAT YOUR DIAGNOSIS IS CORRECT?

Your doctor may be 100 percent sure of what you have. On the other hand, he may have some doubts, but this may be the diagnosis that best fits your symptoms. Ask the doctor if there are other signs or symptoms you should be looking for that will either confirm or refute his diagnosis.

## IF YOU'RE NOT SURE OF THE DIAGNOSIS, HOW CAN YOU BE SURE THAT THE TREATMENT WILL WORK?

In some cases, the doctor suggests a treatment, but isn't sure that it is going to work. It could be a diagnosis by process of elimination: if I treat you for X and you don't get better, then we can assume you don't have X. If the doctor still can't make a diagnosis, you should seek a second or third opinion.

## ARE THERE ANY ILLNESSES THAT CAN'T BE DIAGNOSED?

New diseases are cropping up all the time, just as there are new cures that are being discovered. There are some diseases that medical science hasn't yet learned how to diagnose.

## IF THAT'S THE CASE, AM I GOING TO DIE FROM IT?

The truth is that many people have conditions that are undefined and undiagnosed, yet they live a relatively normal life for years and years.

Says Dr. Strauss, "We talked before about being chronically fatigued. Some people are tired all the time, and nobody knows why they are tired. They may see dozens of experts, and no one can tell them why they're so tired, and they continue to live normal, albeit tired, lives.

"I've had people come in complaining of pain and swelling in their legs. I examine their legs, and even though they don't look very swollen, I check their circulation and find that it's normal. I check for arthritis, I check for soft-tissue inflammation, and I check for nerve inflammation. Everything seems to be normal, yet the complaints continue. I may never figure out where these symptoms and pains are coming from. There are a great many conditions in life that medical science is unable to diagnose, but most won't affect your longevity."

\*    \*    \*

## IS THERE LITERATURE AVAILABLE ON THIS DISEASE OR CONDITION SO I CAN READ UP ON IT AT HOME?

The doctor may have some literature right there in the office, or she may know where you can get it. There may be a medical library nearby. Or she may be able to photocopy some material and give it to you.

# SECTION 5

# SMART QUESTIONS TO ASK ABOUT TREATMENTS AND MEDICATION

Several years ago, my husband went to see a doctor about some digestive problems he was having. I sat in as the doctor suggested a course of action. One of the things he said was, "You can't eat too many green leafy vegetables."

As we were preparing dinner that evening, my husband opened the cupboard and took down a large wooden bowl. I watched in disbelief as he began to make a huge spinach salad.

"What are you doing?" I asked. "The doctor told you not to eat any green leafy vegetables!"

"No he didn't," by husband replied. "He told me I couldn't eat too many—that means no amount is too much."

Which one of us was right? We both heard the doctor say the same words, yet we came up with totally opposite interpretations.

Unfortunately, this is common in everyday communication. When the subject is your health, however, miscommunication can have disastrous results.

You can use questions to probe and clarify. If the doctor says,"You can't have too many onions," ask him to clarify his statement. Ask, "What exactly do you mean by that?"

If the answer is, "I mean you should limit your intake of onions," probe further. Ask, "How many onions can I have?" Keep asking questions until you get a specific answer.

It's important that you get specific answers when discussing treatments and medications. You can use the questions in this section as the place to start. Keep asking probing questions until you're sure you clearly understand the doctor's recommendations.

## WHAT IS THE TREATMENT FOR THIS ILLNESS OR CONDITION?

An even better question might be: "Doctor, how are we going to take care of this condition?" Notice that I say "we." Both you and the doctor must be active participants in your treatment. In fact, often, you play the major role in the treatment of your illness.

There are many different types of treatment available (medication, physical therapy, extended rest and relaxation, etc.), however, not all of them apply to every illness. Whatever the prescribed treatment, it will not work unless you agree to follow instructions.

## ARE THERE ANY ALTERNATIVE TREATMENTS AVAILABLE?

If you are extremely resistant to the form of treatment your doctor recommends, it will probably not help you get better. In some cases, there may be only one course of action for you to follow. In many cases, however, there are choices you can make about how you want to deal with your situation.

Usually, there are many alternative treatments for any one particular problem. Consider alcoholism, for instance. Some doctors prescribe a drug called Antabuse (disulfiram), which is taken on a regular basis. If you drink alcohol while you're taking Antabuse, the combination of the two substances causes a severe reaction. Knowing that the reaction is going to occur is enough to keep some people from drinking.

Another type of treatment for alcoholism is emotional support groups, such as Alcoholics Anonymous. Or you could go into a hospital, where they feed you intravenous fluids and Librium (chlordiazepoxide). There are also "natural" treatments that involve strict diet and exercise to put your system in proper synchronism with the environment, on the theory that this will reduce your desire for alcohol.

Each individual will respond to each of these treatments differently, and this is just one of many diseases that can be treated in a variety of ways.

## IS MEDICATION THE BEST WAY TO TREAT THIS PROBLEM?

Both doctors and patients often use medication as the first response to solving a problem. We've been conditioned by our "immediate gratification" society to want something that will work quickly and painlessly—even if it's not the best solution.

Doctors would love to be able to take care of patients by saying, "Here, take this pill. It will make you better." There is a notion that the easiest, most convenient way of treating the disease is always the best. However, the easiest and most convenient way is not always the most effective—and may, in fact, be extremely damaging.

An example of this is drug addiction. The easiest way to treat pain is to give the patient a narcotic. It's easy, and it gets rid of the pain—until your system becomes adjusted to the narcotic and your pain returns worse than ever. Not only are you then saddled with the original problem, but you've also become addicted to the narcotic.

Never take anything without knowing exactly what it is that you're taking and why you are taking it. Very often, we're so anxious to 'take a pill and be cured' that we don't pay attention to the dangers of becoming overmedicated.

It's possible that drugs are the best or the only answer for your particular problem; however, there may be alternatives to taking prescription medication. If you want to reduce the amount of drugs in your life, research other forms of treatment.

It's not fair to blame doctors for all the overmedication of our society. Dr. Strauss gives this example: "Patients often insist that they receive a prescription. One common example of this has to do with viral upper respiratory infections. These infections are not bacterial infections and so should not be treated with antibiotics. Yet patients often demand the medication, because they think that antibiotics are the cure for all infections. Patients do get better, not as a result of taking the antibiotics, but because they would have gotten better anyway. Your best bet may be to do what your grandmother told you to do: drink lots of hot tea with lemon, gargle with salt water, and try to get more rest."

## EXACTLY WHAT IS THIS MEDICINE YOU'RE PRESCRIBING?

Doctors are usually very happy to talk about medicines, so there shouldn't be any problem with getting the answer to this question.

It's very important that you know exactly what kinds of medication you have been advised to take. If you're in an emergency situation, for instance, you may be asked what you're currently taking. "Mixing" medications can cause severe reactions and the emergency room physician will be cautious about giving you any new medication until he knows what you're already taking. Precious time could be wasted while you try to find out what your present medication is called.

If you change doctors, you'll also need to be able to tell the new doctor what medications you've been taking and for how long.

## WHY IS THIS MEDICINE BEING PRESCRIBED FOR THIS PARTICULAR PROBLEM?

What you're asking, in more formal terms, is, "What are the indications for this medicine?" In other words, what is this medicine used for and how does it work? Is it killing bacteria? Or is it just killing pain?

## WHAT ARE THE CONTRAINDICATIONS TO TAKING THIS MEDICATION?

There are some medications that some people cannot take under any circumstances. This is called absolute contraindications to their use. For example, if you are allergic to penicillin, then under no circumstances can you take penicillin.

There are other drugs that have relative contraindications—which means that you may take them under certain conditions, but not under others. For instance, a drug might be relatively harmless under normal conditions, but cause severe adverse reactions when taken by a person who has a high level of alcohol.

## WHAT ARE THE POSSIBLE ADVERSE REACTIONS TO OR SIDE EFFECTS OF TAKING THIS DRUG?

If you look at the *Physician's Desk Reference* (these books are available to the general population, by the way), you can see that for any given drug, there is anywhere from a half-page to two pages listing precautions and adverse reactions; the latter range from anxiety and insomnia to teratogenicity, which is the harming of the fetus during pregnancy.

There are cautions regarding the effect the drug might have on labor and delivery; whether or not the medicine will interfere with nursing mothers; whether or not the medicine will interact with other medicines. It's important to ask this question, and it's equally important that you let the doctor know whether you are pregnant, are nursing a child, have any allergies, or are taking any other medications.

## WHAT IS THE LIKELIHOOD THAT I WILL EXPERIENCE SIDE EFFECTS FROM THIS DRUG?

If a side effect of a drug is known to be a low-grade headache, does that mean you should expect to get a headache? Does it mean that most people get headaches? Or that 0.1 percent of the people who take this drug get headaches?

If only a very low percentage of people experience side effects from the drug, you may decide to take it. If the percentage is high, however, you'll have to decide whether the benefits are worth the risk.

## DO YOU HAVE ANY LITERATURE AVAILABLE ON THIS MEDICINE?

Many doctors have brochures on medications they frequently prescribe. This gives you the opportunity to read and study the adverse reactions that are more likely to occur and also some of the uncommon adverse reactions. Once again, it's important for you to know what kind of problems you might expect and to be prepared for their occurrence.

Dr. Strauss adds, "I have some patients with whom I am reluctant to discuss complications. If I tell them about certain complications, they'll develop those complications. If you're the sort of person who is easily influenced, then you might think twice about the things you read.

"Usually, what I tell patients about adverse reactions is, 'If you start taking this medicine and don't like the way you're feeling, assume that the new medication is the cause. Stop taking it and call me immediately.'"

## WILL THIS MEDICINE MAKE ME DROWSY?

Dr. Strauss explains: "There are certain medicines that cross the blood-brain barrier—the barrier that protects the brain from harmful chemicals that run through the blood. If you want to fight an infection in the central nervous system, for example, you'll want to use a drug that can cross this barrier.

"Many antihistamines also get through the blood-brain barrier. They make you sleepy because they have sedative properties. If you want to remain functional while taking an antihistamine, you want to use one of the newer ones that are partially blocked by the blood-brain barrier and so don't put you to sleep."

## WHEN SHOULD I TAKE THIS MEDICINE?

This question is a definite candidate for probing and clarifying. It's very important that you ask for a specific answer. As Dr. Strauss relates, "I once had a patient who asked me when he should take a prescribed medicine, and I said that he should take it at night. The patient then told me, 'I work the night shift, from 11:00 p.m. to 7:00 a.m., so I don't sleep at night when other people sleep. I sleep during the day.'

"The medicine I was giving that patient was an antidepressant with heavy sedative properties. I was assuming that he went to bed at night like most people do, but I was incorrect. When I was given the correct information, I prescribed that the medication be taken at 7:00 a.m., which was correct under those circumstances."

## HOW OFTEN SHOULD I TAKE THIS MEDICATION?

This information often can be found on the bottle's label. Still, it's a good idea to ask your doctor, because the druggist may have made a mistake in the labeling instructions. This doesn't happen often, but it is possible.

Once again, be specific. If you're told, "Take this medicine three times a day," ask, "Exactly what times do you mean?"

There are certain medicines that need to be taken at certain times of the day. One example in this category is birth control pills, which are most effective if you take them at the same time, within an hour, each day. If you don't, the chances of getting pregnant are increased significantly.

## EXACTLY HOW SHOULD I TAKE THIS MEDICATION?

Are there any special instructions that go along with this medication? For instance, tetracycline—which is an antibiotic—should not be taken with food; it should be taken on an empty stomach. There are other medicines that should be taken with food, such as those arthritis pills that tend to be irritating if they're taken on an empty stomach.

## HOW LONG DOES IT TAKE FOR THIS MEDICATION TO TAKE EFFECT?

You're asking this question because you want to know, "Am I going to feel better right away, in two days, or in two weeks?"

For instance, antidepressants can take anywhere from two to four weeks before they are effective. Nonsteroidal anti-inflammatory drugs—which are used for arthritis—frequently take days or weeks before you feel their effects. Other medications, such as antihistamines, take effect rather rapidly.

## HOW DO I KNOW IF THIS MEDICINE IS NOT WORKING?

If the doctor says that you should be feeling better within a week to ten days, and ten days pass and you don't feel any better, the medicine is probably not working. At this point, you should call your doctor and inform her that there has been no change in your health or that your symptoms have not gone away. She may ask you to come in for another office visit or she may prescribe a different medication over the phone.

## WILL THIS MEDICATION INTERACT WITH ANY OF THE MEDICATIONS I AM CURRENTLY TAKING?

It's vitally important that you let your doctor know

what medications you are currently taking whenever a new drug is being prescribed. Two drugs that are very safe when taken separately may be very dangerous when taken together.

Not all interactions are known to the doctor, simply because there are so many drugs out there and so many possible combinations of drugs. It also depends on the individual who is taking the drug. Some people may react and others may not. The doctor may not be able to give you a completely certain answer. It's your responsibility to let the doctor know if you're experiencing adverse reactions and to stop taking the medicine immediately.

Says Dr. Strauss, "I recently had a patient who was taking amoxicillin (a type of penicillin) for an ear infection and congestion in the sinus tract, so I added a decongestant antihistamine. As far as I knew, the antihistamine and the amoxicillin would not interact harmfully. The patient had taken both medicines before, although not at the same time.

"When the patient took them together, he became nauseated and dizzy. When we switched to a different antihistamine, the patient had no further problems. I can't say for sure that the problem was a reaction to the two drugs, but we're not going to try it again to find out. We'll make a note on his chart that this happened and remain aware of it in the future."

## DO I NEED TO TAKE THE ENTIRE BOTTLE OF PILLS OR CAN I STOP TAKING THE MEDICINE WHEN I FEEL BETTER?

You might be tempted to stop taking your medication when the outward symptoms disappear. But certain infections, for instance, take longer to disappear than the symptoms they cause. Thus you should keep taking the medication until the amount prescribed has been used up.

"Strep throat is a perfect example of this situation," says Dr. Strauss. "The treatment for this illness is at least a ten-day supply of penicillin. After two days of medication, the symptoms usually disappear. Many people then stop taking the penicillin. A day or two later, the strep throat returns because the bacteria have not been killed off."

There are other drugs, such as nonsteroidal anti-inflammatory drugs, that you may take only as needed. For instance, if you have a sprained ankle and you have severe swelling and inflammation, you may get better before you finish taking all the pills in the bottle. Once your ankle is better, there's no need to continue taking the medication.

## HOW SHOULD I STORE THIS MEDICINE?

Do I need to refrigerate this medicine? Do I need to keep it in a dry place? Do I need to keep it at a certain temperature? How long can I keep it before it goes bad? How long will it be before I need a refill?

If you don't know the answers to these questions, you can find yourself out of medicine, with expired medicine, or with ineffective medicine. Medicine will do you no good once it becomes inert or inactive.

Make sure that you know how, where, and how long to keep your medication.

## I HAVE CHILDREN IN THE HOUSE. WHAT PRECAUTIONS DO I NEED TO TAKE?

You need to take precautions similar to those you would take with any toxic substances you may have around the house—keep them out of reach, in locked cabinets or on high shelves. Most pharmacists offer pill containers with childproof caps. (Unfortunately, they're often peopleproof caps and are difficult for anyone to open.)

You should also be aware that there are certain substances around the house that have a high overdose probability. It's not unusual, for example, for children to grab a bottle of chewable vitamins and chug a bunch of them down. Don't be fooled by products that seem harmless. Keep anything children are able to pop in their mouths tightly sealed and out of reach.

## WHAT SHOULD I DO IF MY CHILD SWALLOWS SOME OF MY PILLS?

The usual answer is, "Go to the emergency room." You should also keep the phone number of your local poison control center near the telephone. Keep a bottle of syrup of ipecac in the house. You may be told to make your child vomit and the ipecac is used for this purpose.

## I CAN'T READ THIS PRESCRIPTION. WILL THE PHARMACIST BE ABLE TO?

Physicians are notorious for having illegible handwriting. Make sure that the pharmacist will be able to understand the prescription. Believe it or not, pharmacists often have to call the doctor and say, "Hey, doctor, what did you write here?" A lot of people make jokes about doctors' scribblings, but joking is not going to help your health care.

## WHAT IS YOUR POLICY ON REFILLING PRESCRIPTIONS OVER THE PHONE?

The answer to this will probably depend on the medication. In some instances, the doctor will have no problem with calling the pharmacy and authorizing a refill. At other times, she may insist that you come in to the office before she will authorize more medication.

## WHAT PHARMACY DO YOU RECOMMEND?

One reason for asking this question is that after being exposed to different pharmacies, doctors often have a feel for which pharmacy is more interested in serving the public—that is to say, which pharmacists care the most and go out of the way for patients. Some will deliver; some stay open longer; some stay open at unusual hours. Sometimes you will find a pharmacist who will get out of bed to serve an after-hours patient.

## DO YOU HAVE ANY SAMPLES OF THIS MEDICATION THAT YOU CAN GIVE ME?

Every day, sales representatives from different pharmaceutical companies visit doctors' offices, and they often leave small quantities of their drugs for the doctors to dispense to patients. The theory behind this is that once the doctor discovers how effective this particular drug is, he'll continue to prescribe it.

Since the samples are free to the doctor, he can give them to his patients at no cost. He thus could save you money by giving you some of the sample drugs he has in his office.

## CAN I USE A GENERIC BRAND OF THE MEDICATION YOU'VE PRESCRIBED?

There is some controversy over whether generic and trade-name medicines are equally effective. The evidence seems to indicate that some generics are just as effective as proprietary drugs and some are less effective. It depends on the particular drug.

Generic drugs are usually less expensive, and so which you will want to buy depends on the efficacy of the generic drug as compared with the trade-name product. Ask your doctor which is more effective. She may have had patients who took both the trade-name and the generic drug and have noticed a difference. If not, check with the pharmacist. If you don't get a satisfactory answer from either, you can call the drug companies, ask them to send you literature, and make your own comparisons.

## ARE THERE ALTERNATIVE THERAPEUTIC MEASURES THAT CAN BE HELPFUL FOR THIS PARTICULAR PROBLEM?

Diet and/or exercise can often be used along with, or in place of, medication. Some people would rather focus on diet than take pills. For example, there are pills that can lower your blood sugar if you're hyperglycemic (diabetic). If you don't want to take pills, you might decide that you will work extra hard at maintaining the American Diabetes Association diet, which, if followed properly, can also lower your blood sugar.

There are some forms of treatment that allow you to exercise your way back to health. Using the example of diabetes again, it's a well-known fact that people can use exercise regimens (along with a reasonable diet) to maintain their blood sugar at a relatively normal level.

## DOES THE EXERCISE ROUTINE HAVE ANY ADVERSE EFFECTS? IF SO, HOW DO I KNOW THAT THEY ARE OCCURRING?

If you are just starting an exercise program, there are

certain precautions that must be taken. For instance, many people who start a jogging program wind up slowly destroying their knees as a result of inadequate preparation and instruction regarding warming up, proper footwear, and proper methods of running.

## HOW DO I KNOW IF THIS TREATMENT IS HURTING ME?

Sometimes it's difficult to know one type of pain from another. You may not actually know whether the pain that you're experiencing—in exercise, for example—is a positive pain or a negative pain.

Exercising can produce some muscle soreness, which is considered a positive pain. However, certain exercises can cause arthritis to develop, which is a negative pain. The arthritis occurs because the muscles are not ready to sustain the skeleton through the exercise routine. As a result, the skeletal system takes the brunt of the stress and deteriorates at the joints, causing arthritis.

Dr. Strauss adds: "Everyone feels pain differently, and it's difficult to describe pain to someone else. People most frequently describe ulcer pain as a burning sensation. Yet I've had patients come in with the same ulcer problems and describe the pain as more of a stabbing sensation. Chest pain, associated with cardiovascular diseases, has a wide range of descriptions—everything from stabbing, to pressure, to burning, to aching.

"You're the best judge of whether or not something is harmful for you. If you experience intense or recurring pain, stop what you're doing and have the doctor check it out."

## WHAT DO I DO IF I'M EXERCISING PROPERLY AND I'M NOT GETTING ANY BETTER?

The best thing to do is to stop what you're doing, call the doctor, and go back for a reevaluation of the problem and the treatment. If your sprained ankle or lower back is not responding to suggested exercises, let the doctor know you are unhappy with the treatment. If you don't, she can't be held fully responsible for the fact that things aren't going well.

## I'M FEELING MUCH BETTER. DOES THAT MEAN I AM BETTER?

This is a difficult question to answer. The example used earlier about the strep throat shows that feeling better is not always an indication of health.

You also need to be careful when taking medication for pain relief. The medication may cause you to feel better, although the problem has not been relieved. It's easy to become dependent, for your own comfort, on these medicines.

## WHAT'S THE DIFFERENCE BETWEEN DEPENDENCY AND ADDICTION?

Dr. Strauss explains: "If a person is addicted to a substance, then it is the substance itself that the person craves. However, you can be dependent on a substance and not actually crave that substance; you can crave the relief that it provides.

"Patients who are medicated for chronic pain usually become dependent on the substance to provide relief from the pain. They don't get 'high' from taking these drugs, but simply experience a diminishment of pain. However, they also experience a diminishment of mental functioning and other adverse affects associated with narcotics. This is different from the actual physical and emotional highs usually experienced by people who are addicted to drugs."

## IF I START TO TAKE A NARCOTIC, DOES THAT MEAN I'M GOING TO BECOME ADDICTED TO IT?

This should be discussed when any narcotic is prescribed. My friend Sheila was having trouble sleeping. She asked her doctor for sleeping pills, and he prescribed them. Sheila was soon addicted and couldn't sleep without them.

She didn't see herself as an addictive personality, so she never asked about the danger involved. And she also thought, "If the doctor is prescribing them for me, it must be right to use them."

After several months on the pills, she finally had a long talk with her doctor and began to ask questions about the pills she was taking. Both she and her doctor realized that Sheila had to break this habit immediately.

The importance of asking this question is to be able to discuss your addiction potential and the addiction potential of the particular medicine. This way, any possible problems that you could develop in the way of physical addictions, as well as emotional addictions, can be avoided.

SECTION 6

# SMART QUESTIONS TO ASK ABOUT CONSULTING ANOTHER PHYSICIAN

When should you go to another doctor to get a second opinion? The answer is: whenever you feel you need one. When I was diagnosed with breast cancer and told I would need a mastectomy, I knew it was time for a second opinion—and a third, fourth, and fifth opinion. You should always get at least one other opinion when surgery is recommended. Most insurance companies insist on it.

Also, there are other reasons besides surgery for seeking advice from another physician. If you're not feeling well, and your doctor can't pinpoint the cause, another doctor may be able to aid in the detective work.

At least two people I know had to consult a second physician because their own doctors couldn't make a diagnosis. Eventually, both of these people found out they had Lyme disease. Although the frequency of this disease is rapidly increasing across the country, neither of the original doctors had ever seen a case before.

A second doctor may have had more experience with your problem, or be a specialist in that area. Diseases do not always follow designated textbook lines. Often, a common illness can take an uncommon turn. If your recovery isn't progressing at a reasonable rate, it could be time to get a second opinion.

This section contains questions to ask your primary health care practitioner before you see a consulting physician. Some of the questions are designed to help you decide whether or not you need a second opinion. Others are meant to furnish you with preliminary information about the second doctor. Still other questions need to be asked after you've seen another doctor, to make sure the consultant and your primary care physician are communicating clearly with each other and with you.

## HOW WOULD YOU FEEL ABOUT MY CONSULTING ANOTHER PHYSICIAN?

If you are not satisfied with the diagnosis or treatment you're getting from your doctor, or if your problem is more complicated then you originally anticipated, then this is a perfectly legitimate question. In fact, you are entitled to get a second opinion for any reason.

However, you should know that some doctors feel threatened when the notion of consulting another physician is introduced. You are, in essence, questioning the doctor's autonomy and authority. Physicians can suffer from insecurity with the best of us.

Yet the question must be asked. And it can be asked in a nonthreatening way. Asking this question is less threatening than saying, "I'm not happy with your diagnosis.

I'm going to see someone else." How you approach the subject depends on the relationship between you and your doctor.

In the final analysis, your doctor was trained to be able to know when he needs a second opinion and when he doesn't. And if it's not necessary, the physician should be given the opportunity to explain why it isn't necessary at this point, and when it might be.

## HOW DO *WE* CHOOSE A CONSULTING PHYSICIAN?

Suppose your physician decides that a consultation is going to be necessary. I cannot emphasize enough that you, as the patient, have the right and the responsibility to be a part of the decision-making process; you must stand up for this right. Don't let the doctor make the choice without you.

There are a lot of factors that go into choosing a consulting physician. Some doctors may be more accessible to you than others; you might prefer to see a specialist who is right next door or in the same building rather than to go across town or to another city. You might have someone particular in mind to whom you want to be referred.

On the other hand, you may have heard negative reports about a specific doctor, and if your doctor is thinking of referring you to that person, you have the right to say "No."

## YOU THINK I SHOULD HAVE SURGERY. WHOM WOULD YOU RECOMMEND I SEE FOR A SECOND OPINION?

When you're looking for a second opinion on whether or not to have surgery, it is generally best to ask both a surgeon and another general practitioner.

Surgeons make their money by doing surgery. Therefore, they might be slightly biased in favor of doing surgery. Surgeons do, however, have information that other physicians may not have. Dr. Strauss gives this example: "Suppose you're asking your pediatrician about circumcising your newborn son. This doctor, who has to deal with the occasional complications of circumcision, recommends that you do not have the surgery performed.

"You go to a surgeon for a second opinion. This doctor sees urological problems that arise in adults who haven't been circumcised. The pediatrician might not be aware of the frequency of this kind of problem. If possible, I'd go to another pediatrician as well and see if I could get a consensus of opinions."

## WHAT CAN YOU TELL ME ABOUT THE PHYSICIAN YOU'VE RECOMMENDED?

The same criteria you used for choosing your primary physician are applicable when picking any physician that you will be consulting. Ask the same questions you asked in Section 2 about the doctor's degrees, reputation, location, office hours, background, and how well he communicates with his patients.

## SHOULD I RETURN TO SEE YOU OR SHOULD I RETURN TO THE CONSULTING PHYSICIAN?

Occasionally, a physician will not be clear as to whether you're to follow up with her or to return to see the consulting physician. The best way to find out is to ask.

## HAS THE CONSULTANT RELAYED HIS OPINION TO YOU?

This is a question to ask your primary care physician after you've seen the consulting physician. It is a way to make sure that the two doctors are communicating and that the "right hand knows what the left hand is doing."

## WHAT DID THE CONSULTING PHYSICIAN TELL YOU?

Perhaps the consultant has relayed information to your doctor that he neglected to tell you. Or perhaps he told you something he forgot to tell the doctor. If your information and the doctor's are the same, then you can be satisfied that there is good communication going on.

## THE CONSULTING PHYSICIAN TOLD ME SOMETHING DIFFERENT THAN HE TOLD YOU. HOW DO YOU ACCOUNT FOR THE DIFFERENCE?

Dr. Strauss tells of a patient he had who came back from a consulting physician and said, "The doctor told me I may need surgery in the future, but there's no hurry." The consultant had told Dr. Strauss that surgery should be scheduled within the next few weeks. The problem was that the patient misunderstood the consultant and translated "within a few weeks" into "there's no hurry."

Occasionally, you'll find a significant discrepancy between what you were told (or think you were told) by the consultant and what he told your doctor. Find out what the communication problem is. It's possible that you did not hear or understand correctly what you were told in the consultant's office. It's also possible that there was a miscommunication between the two doctors.

## I FELT VERY UNCOMFORTABLE WITH THE CONSULTING PHYSICIAN. CAN WE FIND ANOTHER AND HOW ARE WE GOING TO DO THAT?

It's important to let your physician know how you feel. If you're so uncomfortable with the consulting physician that you won't follow her advice or don't trust her opinion, then you may want to go somewhere else.

By asking the question in this way, you enlist your doctor in the process of finding another consulting physician. Once again, this allows you and the physician to be partners in advocating your health. Your physician should have no problem with referring you to someone else.

## I DON'T WANT ANOTHER OPINION, I WANT TO SWITCH TO ANOTHER PHYSICIAN. CAN YOU HELP ME DO THAT?

If you're unable to get in to see the doctor when you need to, if you're not communicating well with the doctor, if you don't believe or trust his diagnoses, or if you simply feel that this doctor is not meeting your needs, you may want to switch to another doctor.

This can be a difficult situation, because nobody likes confrontation. And you are saying things no doctor likes to hear—that the doctor is just not helping you.

You may want to phrase it like this: "I like you as a person, but I'm having difficulty with our medical relationship. I've given this a lot of thought and I've come to the conclusion that I have to transfer to another doctor."

This is a lot like a divorce. It's traumatic for both the doctor and the patient, but it needs to be done.

## WHAT IS THE PROCEDURE FOR TRANSFERRING MY RECORDS TO ANOTHER PHYSICIAN?

Usually, transferring records is taken care of by the new physician. Tell the new doctor that you would like to have your records transferred from your previous doctor's office. She will probably ask you to sign a form and then will take care of the rest of the transaction.

Sometimes the new doctor will want to communicate with the old doctor. They may write letters or talk over the telephone. You may want to suggest this to your new doctor, although it is often standard practice.

## IF I SEE ANOTHER DOCTOR IN AN EMERGENCY, HOW CAN I MAKE SURE THAT YOU GET THE INFORMATION YOU NEED TO FOLLOW UP?

You've gone to the emergency room because of a sudden illness. Tests have been ordered; an investigation has been conducted; you've been evaluated. You either have been admitted to the hospital or sent home.

A smart question for you to ask the emergency room doctor is: "How can I make sure that my primary health care physician follows up on this?" The emergency room physician is not going to see you again. If your problem turns out to be chronic (one that needs to be followed up), then you need to ensure that all the proper information is available for your doctor to check on. You don't want the results of the laboratory work and the investigation to get lost.

## HOW CAN I MAKE SURE YOU ARE NOTIFIED IF I'M IN THE HOSPITAL?

If you've been admitted to the hospital after a visit to

the emergency room, be sure to ask the hospital to notify your doctor. She should know where you are so that she can make the necessary arrangements for your care. You don't want to be taken care of by a stranger. You must ask that your doctor be notified and given all the pertinent information.

# SECTION 7

## SMART QUESTIONS TO ASK THE SPECIALISTS

The human body is astounding in its diversity and complexity. Medicine, which was practiced by even the most primitive societies, is continually striving to unravel all of the body's mysteries and to unveil its deepest secrets.

Over the years, physicians and medical researchers began to follow specialized areas of interest. Some were fascinated by babies and small children, some by diseases, some by the inner workings of the mind, and some by conditions that could be treated or cured by surgical procedures.

As discussed in Section 1, the field of medicine now comprises five areas of specialty:

- Internal medicine
- Obstetrics and gynecology

- Pediatrics
- Psychiatry
- Surgery

This section contains questions for you to ask specialists in each of the first four areas. These are, of course, only a small sampling of the questions you could ask these specialists. We could fill a separate book with questions for each.

Because surgery is such a complex issue even for sample questions, that specialty is covered separately in Section 8.

Once again, use the questions in Section 2, "Choosing a Doctor," to select a specialist. Then use the questions in this section, plus any others you can think of, to get information related specifically to your problem.

## SMART QUESTIONS TO ASK AN INTERNIST

### WHAT PREVIOUS EXPERIENCE HAVE YOU HAD IN TREATING THIS PROBLEM?

You want to know if the doctor has seen other patients with the same or a similar condition. Although every patient is different, you may feel comforted to know that this specialist is familiar with your problem and has previously dealt with its symptoms, complications, and treatment.

### HAVE YOU HAD ANY SPECIAL TRAINING TO DEAL WITH THIS PROBLEM?

Like every other specialty, internal medicine is broken down into many subspecialties. In larger urban areas, you can usually choose to see the appropriate subspecialist; for example, a gastroenterologist for stomach problems or a cardiologist for heart trouble.

Smaller communities may have only one internist. If you're having stomach problems and the internist has not had special training in gastroenterology, you could check out neighboring towns or nearby cities to find someone who has.

## HOW WILL MY OVERALL HEALTH AND LIFE-STYLE BE AFFECTED BY THIS ILLNESS?

Will I still be able to function normally? Can I go to work? Can I participate in sports or other physical activities?

You don't want to do anything that will be harmful to your overall health or will slow down your recovery. On the other hand, you don't necessarily have to change everything in your life because you're having a temporary setback.

If the condition is chronic (continuing), then you need to know what kind of long-term adjustments you'll have to make.

## WILL THIS ILLNESS AFFECT MY EMOTIONAL STATE?

Dr. Strauss relates: "I met a man recently who told me a harrowing story. About five years earlier, this man (whom I'll call Harry) had gone through the most difficult period of his life. He couldn't hold a job, he underwent a terrible divorce, and his friends were deserting him right and left. He was having wide mood swings and seemed unable to control himself.

"Harry had a thyroid condition, which affected his hormone levels. He had just begun treatment when all his problems began. It never occurred to him at the time that the mood swings were connected to his illness and treatment.

"The doctor should have warned Harry about the possible effects of this condition, but he didn't. Had Harry asked this question when his condition was first diagnosed, perhaps this time of his life would have been a little easier."

## HOW DO YOU THINK ANOTHER DOCTOR MIGHT APPROACH THIS PROBLEM?

There's no one way to approach any problem. Some doctors may opt for a passive approach and adopt a "wait and see" attitude. They may suggest doing nothing, or rely on diet and exercise until they see how things develop. Other doctors may take an aggressive approach and suggest heavy medication or even surgery.

By asking this question, you get the internist thinking in many different directions, and you also get information on various alternative treatments.

## WHY DO YOU THINK THAT YOUR APPROACH IS THE MOST EFFECTIVE?

Have the doctor spell out the rationale on which he bases his approach. You want to know exactly why he's doing what he is doing, and what he feels it will accomplish.

## DO I NEED ANY IMMUNIZATIONS AS AN ADULT?

Adults usually need vaccines only in special circumstances. If you're traveling overseas, it's advisable to have shots before entering certain countries (check with your doctor about which shots you need and see Section 11 for more questions about travel).

Some physicians recommend that you have a tetanus vaccine every ten years or so; you must have one if you are scratched by a rusty nail or piece of metal. Seniors over the age of 65 who have weakened immune systems are urged to get pneumovax and flu vaccines.

## WHAT IS YOUR OPINION OF A LIVING WILL?

A living will is a statement you sign to the effect that you do not want any extraordinary measures taken to maintain your life in a situation in which you cannot voice a decision, such as a continuing coma or the presence of irreversible brain damage. This is an area of some controversy and requires careful thought on your part.

Internists often deal with "end of life" situations. This doctor's experiences may help you decide how you feel about this issue.

# SMART QUESTIONS TO ASK A GYNE-COLOGIST/OBSTETRICIAN

## WHAT IS A PAP SMEAR?

A Pap smear, named for scientist George Papanicolaou, is essentially the collecting of cervical cells of the uterus. The cervix is the narrow outer end of the uterus that is the exit through which a child is born. By examining these cells under a microscope, one can detect any abnormalities that might indicate cancer.

## IS A PAP SMEAR PAINFUL?

Although they're not usually painful, pelvic exams can be very uncomfortable (especially if you've never had one before). Gynecologists do so many Pap smears and pelvic exams that it's easy for them to become desensitized to what their patients are going through.

The fact is that every woman who asks, "Is this going to be painful?" reminds the doctor that it is more than just a procedure. For the patient, it can be a traumatic event.

## TO WHAT LABORATORY DO YOU SEND YOUR PAP SMEARS? ARE YOU PLEASED WITH THE LAB'S SERVICE AND WITH ITS TECHNIQUES AND INTERPRETATIONS?

The Pap smear is a very potent screening tool: it is low in cost and very effective in preventing cervical cancer, which had previously been one of the worst killers of women in the United States. However, a lot depends on the laboratory processing the smears.

There has been much controversy lately regarding the quality of the laboratories that deal with Pap smears. You can send the same smear to two different labs and have it come back with two different readings, which indicates some variation in the quality of reading and interpreting from lab to lab. Find out the name of the lab your doctor uses. Ask her whether she's satisfied with its service. If this is not an issue about which the gynecologist is concerned, perhaps you will stimulate some thought on her part.

The more questions we ask and the more we push for quality control, the more the laboratories that screen Pap smear tests will take responsibility for the accuracy of their screenings. And the more accurate the labs are, the more effective we will be in detecting cervical cancer.

## HOW OFTEN SHOULD I HAVE PAP SMEARS AND PELVIC EXAMS?

There is no universal agreement as to how often these examinations are necessary. Most doctors recommend that you have your first exam when you reach the age of sexual activity or 18, which ever comes first, and continue to have exams at a rate of anywhere from every one to every three years.

Your family history can influence the frequency of these exams. If the women in your family have had cancer, you should have exams at least once a year. If you've had any abnormal (but not cancerous) Pap smears, you're also a candidate for more frequent exams.

## HOW DO I GET THE RESULTS OF MY PAP SMEAR?

Many times, your gynecologist will say, "If there's any problem, I'll let you know. If you don't hear from me, you can assume that everything's okay." This policy saves the doctor a lot of time, since so many of his patients have lab work done.

However, you may not want to rely on this assumption. You can reply by saying, "Just for my own peace of mind, I'll call you next week to check on the results. When is a good time to reach you?"

## DO YOU WARM YOUR SPECULUM?

A speculum is an instrument which opens the vaginal vault so that a Q-tip can be inserted to collect cervical and vaginal cells. Any woman who has ever had a pelvic exam knows the rationale for asking this question.

## DO YOU HAVE FOOT WARMERS ON YOUR STIRRUPS?

Dr. Strauss says, "I was recently made aware of the fact that foot warmers for the stirrups do, in fact, exist. Stirrups are usually made of hard, cold metal, and women usually have bare feet in them. Self-warmed coverings over these stirrups could make the visit to the gynecologist much pleasanter. As stirrup warmers are fairly new on the scene, many gynecologists may not even know that they are available."

## WHAT CAN YOU TELL ME ABOUT BREAST EXAMS AND MAMMOGRAMS?

Gynecologists should be prepared to discuss all aspects of breast exams and breast cancer prevention.

## HOW OFTEN SHOULD I HAVE A MAMMOGRAM?

A mammogram is an x-ray photo taken of the breast in order to detect cancer. This is another controversial subject in medicine today, and there is disagreement as to how often these x-rays should be done.

The main disagreement is between the American College of Oncologists and the American College of Radiologists. Radiologists (the people who actually take the x-rays) favor more frequent mammograms, often suggesting that they be done yearly. Oncologists (cancer specialists) usually feel that mammograms need not be done quite so often.

## AS A PREGNANT WOMAN, WHAT KIND OF IMMUNIZATIONS AND BLOOD SCREENING TESTS DO I NEED TO BE CONCERNED ABOUT?

These days, various screening measures (including screening for venereal diseases and for diabetes) are being used to protect both mother and child. These include tests for blood incompatibility, in case the mother has one blood type and the father another. A baby with the blood type of the father but growing inside a mother with a different type of blood can experience a negative reaction from the mother's immune system as the mother detects foreign antibodies in her system.

## ARE YOU GOING TO DELIVER MY BABY OR MIGHT IT BE DONE BY ONE OF YOUR PARTNERS?

Frequently, obstetricians are part of a group practice. While you may be assigned to a specific doctor, if you don't go into the hospital on a night when your doctor is on duty, he may not be the one to deliver your baby.

You need to find out—if it's important to you—whether or not the doctor you're seeing now is going to be the one who'll actually do the delivery. If you want to be sure that your doctor will deliver your baby, you may decide you want to go to an obstetrician who is in solo practice.

## WHERE WILL I BE HAVING MY BABY?

Obstetricians can be affiliated with several different hospitals, so you need to find out in which specific hospital you'll be delivering. Be sure you have clear instructions on the fastest routes to your destination. If you live in larger urban areas, have several different routes planned out in case you run into traffic or construction.

## SHOULD I HAVE A SONOGRAM?

A sonogram is a benign procedure in which ultrasound is used to take a "photograph" of an unborn child. It is commonly done at various stages of pregnancy to check on the size of the fetus and get an estimated date of delivery. It's also used to check on the fetal heartbeat, to detect developmental abnormalities, and to determine the sex of the fetus and whether more than one fetus is present.

No sonogram is foolproof, however. So if you've been told to expect a little boy based on the sonogram, don't be too shocked if you end up with a girl after all.

## SHOULD I HAVE AMNIOCENTESIS?

Amniocentesis involves inserting a hollow needle through the abdominal wall and uterus to obtain a sample of amniotic fluid. This procedure is usually done if there is any suspicion of abnormality in the developing fetus.

There are some risks involved, so this is a decision that will have to be discussed and weighed carefully by the parents and the doctor together.

## WHAT DO I NEED TO DO TO PREPARE FOR DELIVERY?

Your obstetrician may have classes or support groups to which he can refer you.

The delivery of a child can be a wonderful experience—if you are mentally and physically prepared. Groups such as Lamaze (which teach expectant mothers and fathers about pregnancy and delivery) go a long way toward preparing the parents. Your obstetrician should have a list of such groups or organizations near you.

## HOW PAINFUL WILL MY LABOR BE?

One of the major problems with pregnancy, and especially with labor, is the fear associated with the experience. Some women, no matter how many children they have, never get over the fear of the pain. Any time you have increased fear and anxiety, the pain will be intensified.

Pregnancy complications are increased in women with increased fear. As the mind and the body interact, they either can interact to produce a relaxed and eloquent delivery or they can result in a problematic, painful delivery. The obstetrician is trained to deal with patients' fears and concerns, as well as with their physical progress.

## IF I DECIDE ON NATURAL CHILDBIRTH, DOES THAT MEAN I WILL GET NOTHING TO MITIGATE PAIN?

Dr. Strauss responds, "The answer really depends on the obstetrician. There are many ways of interpreting 'natural childbirth.' To me, it means that a mother doesn't get anything for pain, except reassurance, and that she is able to experience every aspect of the delivery the way it would be done naturally (completely on her own).

"To other doctors, natural birth simply means having a vaginal birth, and drugs will be used if the doctor and patient agree."

## IS IT POSSIBLE FOR ME TO BE AWAKE DURING CHILDBIRTH WITHOUT EXPERIENCING ALL THAT PAIN?

At present, there are two types of anesthesia you can have and still be awake: Narcotics, such as Demerol, and peripherally acting anesthetics, such as Lidocaine or Novocaine. Narcotics turn off the pain receptors in the brain; the "caines" turn off the pain receptors in the nerve endings.

## WHAT ARE THE RISKS INVOLVED?

If you use a narcotic, there are small risks of over sedation and sometimes even respiratory suppression. Peripherally acting anesthetics can block muscle strength at the same time they block the pain, in which case the muscle contractions of the uterus will not be strong enough and pushing will be more difficult.

## WHEN DO YOU USE PERIPHERALLY ACTING ANESTHETICS?

When labor begins, the cervix is at 0 centimeters dilation, and opens progressively to about 10 centimeters dilation, at which time the baby will proceed out of the uterus through the birth canal. Approximately halfway through this process, at about 5 centimeters dilation, it is usually safe to administer peripherally acting anesthetics.

## WHAT IF I AM IN SEVERE PAIN BEFORE I REACH 5 CENTIMETERS?

Administering narcotics early in the labor process could put you to sleep so that you don't remember the childbirth, it could make labor more difficult, and, in extreme cases, it could suppress the baby's respiration. Doctors try not to use narcotics if they feel the baby will be born within an hour or two.

## WILL I HAVE TO BE PUT TO SLEEP IF I NEED A CESAREAN SECTION?

Not necessarily. If you have an epidural block already in place, that may be sufficient to block the pain.

## IS GENERAL ANESTHESIA EVER USED?

General anesthesia is sometimes used when a Cesarean must be performed quickly and there is not time for an epidural block.

## HOW DO YOU FEEL ABOUT EPIDURALS?

An epidural is a type of regional nerve block in which a tube is inserted into the lower spinal canal around the third lumbar vertebra and an anesthetic is injected into the spinal canal. The anesthetic causes numbing of the entire lower area of the body; therefore, the patient feels no pain during delivery.

Some obstetricians are in favor of and recommend the procedure regularly; others tend to avoid it. Find out where your obstetrician stands on the subject.

## WHAT ARE SOME OF THE POSITIVES AND NEGATIVES ABOUT EPIDURALS?

The positives are, first, that you get to enjoy a relatively painless delivery. Second, relieving the pain enables you to focus more on the birth process and better endure a lengthy labor and delivery.

Epidurals can, however, decrease the mother's ability

to push the baby out because of the muscle laxity from the numbing. They can also lead to headaches and/or lower back pain after the birthing procedure.

## WHAT IS YOUR CESAREAN SECTION RATE?

Some physicians are more prone to performing cesarean sections than are others. If your obstetrician has a high rate of these operations, it means that this is usually his choice at the first sign of trouble. Other obstetricians are not as quick to do a cesarean section. They wait longer to see how things will develop.

Although cesarean sections have improved over the years, they still present a certain amount of risk, as any surgery does. They decrease the risks to the child during a problem delivery, but increase the risks to the mother (of possible infection or excess bleeding).

In the old days, once you had a vertical cesarean section, you couldn't ever have a natural delivery. Today, with the low, horizontal incision, if one child was delivered by a cesarean, natural delivery is still possible for other children.

## WHAT SORT OF ARRANGEMENTS ARE MADE FOR BONDING BETWEEN MY CHILD AND ME AFTER THE DELIVERY?

Some hospitals separate mother and child as if the two were not meant to be together. The child goes to the nursery; Mom goes to her room. And they don't see each other for quite a long time (anywhere from four to six hours; the hospital only brings the babies to the mothers to be fed). However, in other hospitals, the baby is brought to the mother immediately following delivery.

Newer hospitals often have rooming-in facilities, where the baby actually stays with the mother all the time, instead of just at appointed times for feeding. This is a matter of personal preference. Some mothers who have had dramatic deliveries prefer to rest and recuperate for a while. You need to find out what your obstetrician thinks about all these options and what the hospital policy is.

## HOW DO YOU FEEL ABOUT BIRTHING CENTERS? HOW DO YOU FEEL ABOUT DELIVERY AT HOME?

Today there are options as to how and where you can have your children born. Deliveries can be made in the standard hospital setting, they can be done at home, or, in some areas, they can be done in birthing centers.

A birthing center is a place that usually tries to provide a down-home, relaxed, nonclinical setting in which to give birth. It would not be unusual for a birthing center to look like someone's living room or bedroom, except that clamps, suction devices, sutures, and other types of apparatus for aiding in deliveries are kept nearby.

Birthing centers are generally located near a hospital, or sometimes in hospitals themselves, so as to provide adequate coverage in the event of complications during delivery.

Dr. Strauss relates this story about home births: "My last child was delivered at home, and it was a thrilling experience. At 5:00 p.m., my wife, Schrea, started to have labor pains. At 6:00, she informed me about them. At 7:00, I built a nice, comfortable fire in the fireplace (it was December). At 8:00, we started to play a game of chess and at 9:00 she beat me. At 10:00 the contractions got harder, and by 11:00, she had 'spit that baby out.' The birth was completely without complications. Everything was smooth, joyful, and exciting. I wouldn't have traded the experience for anything.

"A midwife was on the scene to take part in the delivery, and she was the one who actually delivered the baby so that I could share in the birth moment.

"The reason I was able to do that with a fair degree of peace of mind was because I had participated in Schrea's previous delivery (in the hospital) and it went without a hitch. When you have a pattern of uncomplicated births, you can generally feel comfortable about doing home deliveries. The fact that I am a doctor, of course, made it easier to justify. Yet I didn't use any of my skills as a doctor during that evening."

## WHAT ARE SOME OF THE DANGERS ASSOCIATED WITH HOME DELIVERY?

"If there's any problem with the delivery, you have to get the mother and child to the hospital, and you have to do it fast," says Dr. Strauss. "If you decide to go with the home delivery, you must be prepared to get to a hospital in case of an emergency or in case a cesarean section needs to be performed.

"I would not advise having your first baby at home (if you have a choice), because there is no precedent for how it will go."

## HOW DO YOU FEEL ABOUT MIDWIVES?

Conventional medicine tends to shy away from midwifery in the delivery of babies. As Dr. Strauss points out, however, "Out here in Kentucky, where obstetricians are not always readily available, midwives were the standard for a long time and are still widely accepted.

"Recently, midwives have had a great deal of difficulty getting malpractice insurance to cover their liability; in some places, they're no longer able to deliver due to increased malpractice insurance rates.

"If you decide you want to go with a midwife, check carefully into her background and experience. Find someone you like and trust. Once again, be sure you are prepared for any emergency that might arise."

## WHAT IS A D&C?

The initials D&C stand for dilation and curettage. It's a procedure designed to remove excess tissue from the uterine wall, which can cause excessive bleeding. The cervical os (the small hole that is the passageway into the uterus) is dilated, or opened, and the curettage (tissue-removing) instrument is inserted. The same procedure can be used for an endometrial biopsy, to determine whether or not there is cancer present.

The danger of this procedure is that too much tissue can be removed and a women's menstrual periods could stop for months, years, or forever.

# SMART QUESTIONS TO ASK A PEDIATRICIAN

## DO YOU HAVE ANY CHILDREN?

It's always easier to relate to a pediatrician if he has had children of his own. That is not to say that a person who has never had children can't be a good pediatrician. You just want to know exactly how well the doctor can understand the problems you or your child or children are having.

## WHAT KIND OF HEALTH MAINTENANCE DO YOU ADVOCATE FOR MY CHILDREN?

There are various types of health maintenance programs for children, starting at the age of two weeks and continuing until the children are no longer in the pediatric age group.

The standard, or traditional, position concerning child health maintenance is the one suggested by the American College of Pediatricians. This includes setting a schedule of immunizations at varying stages of the child's development, measuring the child's growth (height and weight) at certain ages, examining vision and hearing, and periodically checking behavioral status and fine motor, gross motor, and social skills.

A lot of information is available about what to expect from children as they develop. Behavioral factors are examined according to the age of the child. You can ask your pediatrician such questions as, "My baby is six months old. What should she be doing now?" Or, "My baby hasn't started walking yet. Is anything wrong?"

Children develop at their own pace. There may not be anything wrong if your child is not progressing as quickly as some other children of the same age. If there is something wrong, however, you want to become aware of it as early as possible.

## ARE YOU FAMILIAR WITH THE DENVER DEVELOPMENTAL SCALE FOR CHILD DEVELOPMENT?

The Denver Developmental Scale is a set of norms for the gross motor, fine motor, social, and language development of children as they grow. By determining your child's location on this scale, you can gauge his or her progress as compared with other children of the same age.

The use of this scale should enable the pediatrician to tell you what your child should be able to accomplish within a given age range and what you should be expecting your child to do in the future.

## SHOULD I BE BREAST-FEEDING MY BABY?

There are many different factors that go into making this decision, and they should all be discussed with the pediatrician. For one thing, the mother's overall health, as well as the child's, should be taken into account.

This is also a life-style choice. If the mother is working, it may not be practical to breast-feed (although it may still be possible to feed the child breast milk by pumping the mother's milk into a bottle). There are positives and negatives on both sides of this decision.

## AT WHAT AGE SHOULD I INCORPORATE REGULAR FOODS INTO MY CHILD'S DIET?

If I'm not breast-feeding, what kind of formula should I use? When can I start giving my child baby food? When can I start giving my child regular adult food? Are there any foods that should be avoided? Are there any foods that must be included? These are all questions with complicated answers.

"Breast milk is generally considered the most complete food a human being can digest," says Dr. Strauss. "You could live your whole life on breast milk, except that it lacks sufficient iron. However, not every mother is willing or able to breast-feed, and there are many other healthy choices.

"You could spend a week in the grocery store studying baby foods and formulas. Formulas are made of three ingredients: a protein (usually some form of whey), milk sugar (lactose), and milk fat. Children can have allergic reactions to any one of these ingredients. That's why they've now developed formulas that include other kinds of proteins, or are lactose-free, or contain only simple fats and sugars.

"As for baby foods, pediatricians will generally start

kids on rice and grains at five or six months of age. Parents usually start a lot earlier, however. Some children can eat baby foods—or any foods, for that matter—at any age with no problem; others have bad reactions. If your children are frequently sick, especially with diarrhea or bowel problems, food is probably the culprit. Trial and error will tell you what your children can eat and what they can't. I spent a large part of my training in pediatrics residency changing babies' diets."

## HOW PREVALENT ARE ALLERGIES IN CHILDREN?

According to Dr. Strauss, "There are many different opinions about just what allergies are and how to treat them. I believe that just about everybody is allergic to something. Some people may have allergies and never even know it. Others are very sensitive and are highly allergic."

Children often have allergies. Some are caused by foods and some by environmental factors. To determine the cause, pediatricians usually start by eliminating various foods from the child's diet. Children often grow out of many allergies as they get older. But if the allergies persist, you may want to consult an allergy specialist.

## WHAT SORT OF FOODS SHOULD MY CHILD BE EATING?

Nutrition has great bearing on your child's physical development, now and in the future, as the child learns good eating habits.

You're liable to find that different health professionals have different emphases. Some health professionals don't stress nutrition at all, while others feel that it's vitally important to a child's development.

Some doctors feel that children should avoid excess

sugar and that large quantities of sugar can be harmful. You may be advised to watch fat and cholesterol levels, even in young children. There are doctors who recommend feeding your children only organically grown fruits and vegetables. You'll have to weigh your doctor's suggestions against your own philosophy, as well as your child's food preferences (no food is good for a child who won't eat it).

## HOW OFTEN DO YOU RECOMMENDED I BRING MY CHILD IN TO SEE YOU?

The frequency of visits generally corresponds to vaccinations. For example, the polio vaccine and the diphtheria-pertusis-tetanus vaccines are generally given at 2, 4, 6, and 18 months and 4 years of age. At 1 year of age, a tuberculant skin test is done. At 15 months of age, a measles, mumps, and rubella vaccine is given. A new vaccine, the Hemophilus Influenza B (HIB) vaccine, is given between 15 months and 2 years. Recently, the measles, mumps and rubella vaccine has been advocated for 4-year-olds as well.

## DO YOU GIVE CHILDREN IMMUNIZATIONS IN YOUR OFFICE OR DO YOU SEND THEM TO THE HEALTH DEPARTMENT?

Because of the price of immunizations these days, children are often sent to local health departments rather than being given shots in the office of the pediatrician or family physician.

It is usually less expensive to go to the health department, but you may wind up waiting for several hours because of the large numbers of people. Be sure you know the hours and location of the health department, if you choose to go there.

Visit your health department before you make a decision. In some towns, this office is not crowded, the staff is friendly, and the rooms are bright and warm. In other places, the ambience of the health department is not very pleasant, so it may easier on the child to have immunizations take place in the doctor's office.

## WILL YOU BE CHECKING MY CHILDREN'S EYES AND EARS?

According to Dr. Strauss, "The school system generally provides eye and ear examinations. I would suggest, however, that you have these examinations done in the pediatrician's office, even before your children reach school age.

"Vision and hearing tests can now detect abnormalities at an early age. Problems such as amblyopia, which is the lazy eye syndrome, are usually better dealt with before school starts. That way a child doesn't have to wear an eye patch at the same time he or she is becoming adjusted to being in school."

## AT WHAT AGE SHOULD CHILDREN BE TAKEN TO TO THE DENTIST?

If your children have teeth and can sit in one place for more than a few minutes, then you should take them to the dentist. Bringing them in early acclimates them to the dentist's office, which can be a frightening place to a child.

If visits are started early and treated as a fun experience, children are more likely to think of brushing their teeth and going to the dentist as something they enjoy doing.

## WHAT ARE YOUR VIEWS ON TOILET TRAINING?

"The pediatrician should be ready, willing, and able to deal with all behavioral and emotional issues of child development—including toilet training," says Dr. Strauss.

"Toilet training is a complicated issue. Parents often feel social embarrassment. A woman I was speaking to recently told me this was the case when her child, who had never been toilet trained, continued wetting his pants. All sorts of doubts arose in this mother's mind: 'Am I a good mother?' 'Is there something wrong with my child that he continues to wet his pants?' I had to reassure her that she was doing nothing wrong, and that her son was perfectly normal.

"Toilet training is one of the hallmarks of an infant's coming of age. It is the first step toward acclimation into society. The discussion of toilet training—like the discussion of school preparation, of sexuality, of job preference, of marriage, or of parenting—is a major landmark in a human being's life. It is accompanied by a lot of emotion, for both you and your child. Your doctor should be able to help you both prepare for the experience."

## HOW DO I KNOW IF MY CHILD IS ACTING ABNORMALLY?

The best way to find out if your child is acting abnormally is to observe your child's behavior, observe how other children are behaving, and compare the two. If you suspect that your child's behavior does not fall within the norm, then you should discuss the issue with professionals.

Your physician should not be the only person you ask, however, because the doctor won't know how your child acts under normal circumstances—children never act normally when they're in the doctor's office. The pediatrician will probably recommend that you and she consult the significant people in your child's life—your child's teachers, babysitter, or day-care workers—the people that see your child on a daily basis. Then you can compare your child's behavior in all these different places and see if you get a picture of a normally active child.

## CAN I CALL YOU IF I HAVE ANY QUESTIONS? HOW CAN I CONTACT YOU AFTER OFFICE HOURS?

Pediatricians probably receive more calls than any other kind of physician—especially from first-time parents. Children can often develop illnesses, especially high fevers, very rapidly, so be sure you know how to reach your pediatrician and that you keep emergency numbers near the telephone.

# SMART QUESTIONS TO ASK A MENTAL HEALTH PROFESSIONAL

## HOW DO I KNOW WHETHER I NEED COUNSELING?

When you have a problem, it usually helps to talk it out with someone. Counseling can be a great help in many situations. You don't have to be facing major life traumas. We all occasionally get bogged down in everyday life.

If you're considering counseling, you must find someone you trust, someone with whom you can communicate freely.

Asking this question can tell you a lot about the counselor's philosophy—his ideas about the necessity for counseling in general and for you specifically.

## WHAT ARE YOUR QUALIFICATIONS FOR COUNSELING?

As with any other doctor you consult, you want to find out something about the counselor's background and training. Where did she do her training? How large is her practice? How long has she been in practice? How long does the average patient stay with her?

Generally, the more qualifications a counselor has, the more expensive she will be. Therefore, the psychiatrist tends to be more expensive (slightly) than the Ph.D. psychologist, who tends to be more expensive than the master's degree psychologist, who tends to be more expensive than the licensed clinical social worker, and so forth.

A psychiatrist is the only mental health care professional with a medical degree and the only one able to prescribe medication.

## WHAT KIND OF COUNSELING DO YOU DO?

There are many different approaches to counseling, perhaps the most famous of which is Freudian analysis. The Freudian analyst enables you to explore your thoughts and feeling in great depth and to relate them to your past history. This kind of analysis is done over a long period, as you continue providing the analyst with a detailed account of past and present mental and emotional experiences. The analyst tries to discover your unconscious conflicts. He helps you to become aware of, and to resolve, these conflicts.

There are other types of counseling that deal less with the past and the reasons behind your problems and concentrate more on changing and improving current behavior patterns.

These are only two of the many forms of counseling available, and you may want to visit several different people before you decide on the best one for you.

## HOW LONG WILL I NEED COUNSELING?

There is no universal answer to this question. It depends

on your problem and the individual counselor's particular perspective. Some problems, like chronic illnesses, never go away and are dealt with in an ongoing therapeutic process.

There are problems that are quite severe; for example, neurochemical disorders that produce serious conditions such as schizophrenia. Other anxiety disorders, such as those leading to addictive disorders, aren't necessarily permanent, but may have long-term ramifications.

Some stress-induced problems will prove to be short-lived, and can be helped within a few sessions. This is usually a matter for discussion between you and the counselor once the therapy is in progress.

## HOW WILL I KNOW IF THE COUNSELING IS WORKING?

There may not be any crystal-clear indications as to whether or not you're being helped by counseling. Do you feel different from when you began therapy? Are you behaving any differently? Do you see any difference in your attitudes toward work, relationships, or life in general? You should see some changes, even if they seem small or are slow to happen.

These changes can be very subtle. Your friends and family may notice changes before you do. It's also possible that you'll go through a period of getting worse before you get better. Don't give up after only one or two sessions; give yourself a chance to change.

At some point, the issue always arises as to whether to continue with counseling, as to whether it is doing "any good." It's important to let the counselor know when you're feeling dissatisfied with the way the counseling is going, so that any problems can be addressed and rectified.

## DO YOU PRACTICE GROUP THERAPY?

Groups can be very effective in terms of modifying behavior. As the saying goes, if one person tells you that you have a tail, you laugh about it, but if six people tell you you have a tail, you turn your head and look.

## HOW CONFIDENTIAL ARE MY VISITS?

All interactions between health care professionals and their clients are confidential. Even the fact that you see a mental health professional remains confidential.

## ARE YOUR FEES NEGOTIABLE?

Frequently, they are. Often counselors will charge on a sliding scale and will make allowances if you're having financial difficulties.

## HAVE YOU EVER BEEN SUBJECT TO ANY DISCIPLINARY ACTIONS BY THE STATE, LOCAL, OR FEDERAL AUTHORITIES FOR ANY REASON?

If you have any suspicions about your counselor, you can check with your state or local board of health or medical association.

If the counselor has had any disciplinary actions taken against him, find out exactly why. Then you can decide whether to stop seeing this particular person.

SECTION 8

# SMART QUESTIONS TO ASK WHEN SURGERY HAS BEEN RECOMMENDED

In some ways, the human body is amazingly resilient. People have been known to survive the worst accidents and the most devastating illnesses. The human body is also amazingly delicate. A slight twist of an ankle can cause intense pain and take weeks to heal. A small cut can sever a nerve and cause numbness or paralysis.

Any kind of surgery, even minor surgery, involves a certain amount of risk. It should never be undertaken without a great deal of thought and consideration.

There are basic questions that need to be answered before any surgery is done:

- Why do I need surgery?
- How will surgery improve my condition?
- What will happen if I don't have surgery?

**123**

•What are the risks involved?
•Do the risks outweigh the benefits?

You should not even entertain the idea of having surgery unless you have clear, complete answers to all of these questions.

These are not, by any means, the only questions you should ask. This section contains many more, and I'm sure you'll be able to think of others. Ask them now—before you go into the hospital, before you have the operation.

Just the thought of surgery makes everyone nervous. Write your questions down; write the answers down. Have someone accompany you to the surgeon's office. Go back again with more questions. Do whatever it takes to ensure that you have all the necessary information.


## WHY DOES SURGERY NEED TO BE DONE?

What is wrong with me and how is surgery going to improve it? As stated earlier, no matter how "simple" the surgery is, there are always risks involved, so this is never a matter to be taken lightly.

There are no guarantees, either, so thinking that surgery will be the definitive answer to your problem may be unwise.

"There are cases where surgery is done on a somewhat speculative basis," explains Dr. Strauss. "Take appendicitis, for example. The doctor is presented with a patient who has pain of an unknown origin in the lower-right-hand side of his abdomen. Fifty percent of the people who are taken to surgery with right-lower-quadrant pain will turn out to have normal appendixes. So why do surgery? The answer is that it is done because the signs of appendicitis are so varied and vague. If you waited until you were absolutely sure it was appendicitis (and sometimes you never really know until after the surgery has taken place), it could be too late.

"Surgeons have decided that it is better to operate and find that you have a normal appendix than to wait and find that your appendix has ruptured.

"Other surgeries are based on more positive diagnoses. For example, gallbladder disease can usually be clearly diagnosed using a sonogram to see if there are any stones, along with an oral cholecystogram. (The patient swallows a pill containing dye and then an x-ray is taken. If the dye shows up in the gallbladder, the bladder is functioning. If no dye appears, the gallbladder is not functioning.) On the basis of these tests, you can make the decision to operate, and know that after surgery the patient is going to feel better."

## TO WHAT EXTENT IS SURGERY GOING TO IMPROVE THINGS?

Dr. Strauss explains, "Some surgery will entirely remove, or cure, the problem. In the gallbladder disease discussed earlier, for example, the removal of the gallbladder also removes the problem (you don't need your gallbladder to survive, just as you can live without your tonsils or appendix).

"Other surgeries are not so clear-cut. Suppose you have arthritis of the knee and are presented with the option of having a joint replacement—having your knee replaced with a prosthesis (a synthetic joint). What's going to happen as a result of removing the old joint and putting in the new, plastic joint?

"Prior to surgery, you've been living with intense pain, which has severely limited your ability to get around. What you should know is that after surgery, you will still have pain and you will still have limitations. The condition will be improved, but not 100 percent.

"Plastic surgery is an area where patients often have unrealistic expectations about the results of the surgery. Some patients are disappointed when surgery doesn't make them look picture perfect."

So it's important to ask just how the surgery will improve your situation and how it will not.

## WHAT WOULD HAPPEN IF I DIDN'T HAVE SURGERY?

If I don't have surgery, will I definitely get worse? Or is there a possibility that I will get better on my own? This is still the age of miracles where anything can happen. A person with terminal cancer can miraculously get better. It doesn't happen very often, but it does happen.

The choice of whether or not to have surgery ultimately remains with you. So you need to know what is likely to occur if you choose not to have surgery.

Sometimes, it's a close call—that is, the results of surgery may not significantly improve your condition. Dr. Strauss again: "I have a friend who has coronary artery disease. He had a coronary angiogram (in which dye is run through the coronary arteries), which showed significant blockage. He was then presented with the option of having surgery.

"The surgeons weren't able to assure my friend that he would definitely live longer and have a higher quality of life if he had the operation. He elected not to have it done. He's now doing very well, although he's careful about his diet and exercise. In this situation, the benefit of having surgery was not strong enough for my friend to choose that option.

"In other circumstances, there might be a definite negative outcome if surgery is not done. Let's use diabetes as an example again. Suppose there is an infection in your leg. Often, a diabetic infection can spread very rapidly and gangrene can set in. There is a great deal of pain and a danger that your whole body can be affected.

"The options are fairly clear as the gangrene is spreading up your leg. If you don't have the leg removed, you can't expect to live very long. In this situation, if the surgery is declined, the outcome is predictably bad. This is a case where knowing what will happen if the surgery is not done would convince you to make a positive choice."

## WHAT ARE THE RISKS OF THIS SURGERY?

This is a question that should always be asked. If this is a serious surgical procedure, there can be serious risks. And some of these risks may cancel out the need for the surgery. Dr. Strauss reports that he's had many patients who have decided, because of their failing physical health, that surgery would not be worth the gain and that they might as well let well enough alone.

An example of this is an 86-year-old man who was in good mental health but had serious gallbladder disease. There was a question of whether or not his gall-bladder should be taken out. He decided that, because of past problems with cardiac disease and his general state of debilitation, he didn't want to go through surgery at this point. In this case, the risks of surgery under the circumstances would have been too high in his view.

If you have any questions about the risks involved in surgery, you can ask someone to give you a preoperative evaluation—in other words, to check your overall health and give an opinion as to how you would stand up to the surgery. Usually, your primary health care physician will do that.

## DO THE RISKS OF THIS SURGERY OUTWEIGH THE NECESSITY FOR IT?

Don't think that the doctor will always recommend

surgery, especially if the risks are high. Remember that it is not in the doctor's interest to lose patients.

You need to know all the pros and cons so that you can make an educated decision. Benjamin Franklin had a very good method for making hard choices. He would take a sheet of paper and draw a vertical line down the center. A the top of the right side, he would write the word "Yes." On the left, he would write the word "No." Then he'd list all the positives on the right and all the negatives on the left. If there were more entries in the right-hand column, he'd make a "Yes" decision. If the left side was longer, the answer would be "No." You can do the same thing with all the pros and cons of the surgery involved. It will give you a clear visual image of both sides of the argument and can help you make your decision.

## CAN YOU DESCRIBE THE SURGERY TO ME IN DETAIL?

There are many reasons for asking this question. If you go to another physician, it will be important for you to be able to describe the surgeries you've had in the past.

Another reason is so that you can be a participant in what goes on. You are more than just an interested bystander. It's your body and your health. Asking the doctor to go over the procedure indicates that you're an intelligent person, that you're interested in what happens to you and why. It creates a bond between you and the physician.

Also, what happens during surgery is really very interesting. Knowing the details of your surgery may give you additional insight into how the body functions and what kind of "miracles" surgeons can perform to keep you healthy.

Medicine is a fascinating science. You'll be missing a golden opportunity to learn something about yourself and about medical science if you don't find out what happens during surgery and how your body is changed by it.

## DO YOU HAVE A BROCHURE THAT EXPLAINS THE SURGERY I'M TO UNDERGO?

Even if your surgeon has explained the procedure to you, it's good to have it in writing so that you can study it on your own. Sometimes, when you're in the surgeon's office, the doctor or the setting can be intimidating and you don't hear everything that's said to you. If you can, get a brochure, take it home, and read it when you have more time to digest the information.

## CAN THIS PROCEDURE BE DONE ON AN OUTPATIENT BASIS?

Outpatient surgery means that you come in, have the procedure done, and go home, all in the same day. Several procedures that used to be performed on an inpatient basis, including tonsillectomies, hernia repairs, and tubal ligations, are now often done on an outpatient basis. There are even some major procedures—such as cardiac catheterization (which is not actually surgery, but does entail a high amount of risk)—that also can be done as outpatient surgery. Insurance companies encourage outpatient procedures whenever possible, because it decreases the hospital costs they would normally have to cover.

Find out if being an outpatient is the best option for you, even if it is available. A few years ago, I had a D&C done, and was told I could choose to stay overnight in the hospital, or to go home that day. Luckily, I chose to remain in the hospital. I had a bad reaction to the anesthetic and needed the night in the hospital. Before deciding, ask what complications can arise from the procedure and what the likelihood is that they will occur.

*   *   *

## WHAT IS MEANT BY THE TERM "EMERGENCY SURGERY"?

Some surgeries are done because there is no other choice. For example, if a person has been in an accident or has a problem that is severe and appears to be life-threatening, the surgeon has to act right away in order to save the patient's life. Any situation of this type is known as emergency surgery.

## WHAT IS MEANT BY THE TERM "ELECTIVE SURGERY"?

There are some surgeries that need to be done, but do not have to be done immediately (removing certain benign tumors, for example). Other surgeries, such as plastic surgeries for purely cosmetic reasons, don't have to be performed at all, and it's the patient's choice to have such surgery done. These surgeries are called elective surgeries.

## WHAT IS MEANT BY THE TERM "INFORMED CONSENT"?

Before surgery is performed you will be asked to sign statements to the effect that you understand and approve of the procedure. Witnesses have to be present to make sure that you do understand and that you are mentally alert.

Hospitals and surgeons are fearful of being sued, so they try to be as explicit as possible about the procedure, the risks, and the possible outcome. It stands to reason that you should be interested as well.

## I'M TAKING MEDICATION AT HOME NOW. WILL I CONTINUE TO RECEIVE THAT MEDICATION IN THE HOSPITAL?

Ask your doctor if the medication(s) you are taking at

home will be continued during your hospital stay. You want to make sure that the treatment you're receiving as an outpatient will continue as an inpatient. If you are taking medicines at home but are not receiving them in the hospital, you should find out why.

It's possible that it's the same medication, but in a different form—because it's produced by a different company or is a generic brand. If you're not sure, ask!

## WILL I BE RECEIVING ANY OTHER MEDICATIONS WHILE I'M IN THE HOSPITAL?

I wouldn't be here today writing **this** book if I hadn't once asked a Smart Question.

Several years ago, I was hospitalized for a fever of unknown origin. I am allergic to penicillin, and this was noted on all my medical charts and records. I even wear a bracelet to indicate my allergy. Yet one morning a nurse walked in prepared to give me an injection. If I hadn't quickly asked what was in the needle, I would never have left the hospital alive. Check with your doctor to find out what medications have been ordered for you and ask "What is that?" every time someone wants to give you a pill or injection.

## WHAT IS THE ANESTHESIOLOGIST'S ROLE IN THE SURGERY?

The anesthesiologist is one doctor you may not see very much. You will receive a bill from him, however, and it can be surprisingly high. The anesthesiologist pays enormous malpractice premiums because he is actually in charge of your well-being during and immediately following surgery—and is often the first one blamed if anything goes wrong.

He will visit you before your operation and do an evaluation to make sure that you are an appropriate candidate for surgery, provided the attending physician hasn't done this already.

## WHAT QUALIFIES THE ANESTHESIOLOGIST TO ASSESS WHAT KIND OF RISKS I MIGHT HAVE FOR SURGERY?

The anesthesiologist is a doctor who has gone through four years of medical school and a three-year residency program specifically designed to teach her to assess how well patients will fare under anesthesia during surgery.

## IS THIS PERSON AN ANESTHESIOLOGIST OR A NURSE ANESTHETIST?

An anesthesiologist is a doctor who has done a residency in anesthesiology. A nurse anesthetist is a nurse who has spent time studying anesthesia under an anesthesiologist.

Nurse anesthetists are usually very good at their jobs and are well trained in terms of providing anesthesia. However, if complications arise, it is the anesthesiologist who ends up taking care of you. In some smaller, rural hospitals, the only person available is a nurse anesthetist. When complicated surgery is to be performed, these hospitals "import" an anesthesiologist from a neighboring community.

If you are uncomfortable with the idea of a nurse anesthetist, you may want to go to another hospital.

## WHAT ARE THE RISKS OF ANESTHESIA?

There's always the possibility that the anesthesia will be fatal. Every once in a great while, people just don't wake up from anesthesia. And while the chances of this happening are very remote, the hospital informs every patient of the risk. (Anesthesia is discussed fully in the next section.)

## ARE YOU GOING TO BE TAKING CARE OF ME WHILE I'M IN THE HOSPITAL?

Usually, your physician will tell you if she's not going to be there during your hospital stay—if she's going on vacation or out of town or even taking a few days off. Doctors arrange to have a colleague "cover for them" in their absence. You want to know whom to expect in such a situation.

## WHEN WILL YOU COME TO SEE ME ONCE I AM IN THE HOSPITAL?

Sometimes the physician doesn't get to see you right away. He may not appear until the next morning or the following evening. If you know when to expect the doctor, you won't get angry waiting for him to arrive.

## HOW CAN I GET IN TOUCH WITH YOU WHILE I'M IN THE HOSPITAL?

Usually, the best way to get anything accomplished while you're in the hospital is to ask a nurse. However, your physician may tell you to call her directly from your bedside phone.

## HOW AM I GOING TO FEEL IMMEDIATELY FOLLOWING SURGERY?

Some people wake up feeling horrendous. They can't move; they can't think. They're dizzy; they feel nauseous. These are standard reactions to surgery, so don't be surprised if you experience any or all of them.

Certain surgeries are more difficult than others and may cause more postoperative discomfort. For example, you can expect a lot of abdominal pain after abdominal surgery (even sneezing and coughing can be agony) or a lot of chest pain after chest surgery. After surgery involving the lungs, you can expect pain and/or trouble with breathing. Urological surgeries usually require that catheters be inserted into the bladder, which are a nuisance when you want to move around. Other types of surgery require that you be up and moving around as soon as possible.

## HOW LONG WILL I BE IN THE HOSPITAL?

Many people think that because they're in good physical condition or don't take long to overcome minor illnesses, they'll be able to go home almost immediately following their operation. Some do recover fairly quickly, but most people need the full anticipated recovery time.

Dr. Strauss explains that he's had patients come out of difficult surgery and be able to leave the hospital in just a few days, whereas other patients, less tolerant of pain, were laid up for weeks even though their surgery was relatively minor. So even though it's a good idea to ask this question, the answer you'll get will be the average length of stay for patients who have had similar operations. You may require more time to recover or you may be out of the hospital sooner.

## CAN YOU GIVE ME A DAY-BY-DAY SCHEDULE OF RECOVERY?

How will I feel the first day after surgery? How will I feel the second? What will I be able to do the first day, the second, the third? In general, the answers will depend on you. Some patients recover faster than others.

The physician may be able to tell you what other patients have experienced—how fast the general population recovers. For instance, I was amazed when a relative who had undergone prostate surgery was told by the doctor, "In six weeks, you'll be able to lift a horse." And he was exactly right!

## WHAT ARE SOME OF THE COMPLICATIONS THAT COULD ARISE FOLLOWING THIS SURGERY?

Your doctor can talk to you about some of the problems you might run into and the statistical probabilities of their occurrence. If it's a routine, uncomplicated surgery, then that point should be emphasized. It will be comforting to you and it will make your recovery period easier if you know that this is a surgery associated with low risk.

## HOW WILL I KNOW IF SOMETHING IS STARTING TO GO WRONG?

Suppose you are in the hospital and you're not feeling very well after your surgery. You've been told to expect pain and discomfort. How do you know when what you are experiencing goes beyond the pain and discomfort normally associated with this surgery? How do you know that your pain and discomfort are not associated with a complication of the surgery and that something is in fact going wrong?

The fact of the matter is, you may not know. Don't be afraid to be a "complainer." The physicians and the surgeon will only know that something is wrong if you talk to them about how you're feeling and discuss any pain or discomfort you're having. Your questions help them to monitor your progress and enable them to get a jump on complications, if should they occur.

## DO I NEED TO BE ON A SPECIAL DIET WHEN I LEAVE THE HOSPITAL?

Your doctor may recommend that you be on a special diet when you leave the hospital, either for a short recovery period or as your ongoing daily regimen.

After you undergo certain types of abdominal surgery, for instance, a low-fat diet may be recommended. If you've had some renal (kidney) problems, you may be advised to go on a low-protein diet. You may need to follow an adult diabetic diet or stay away from too much salt and sugar.

## CAN SOMEONE EXPLAIN THIS DIET TO ME IN DETAIL?

Frequently, patients leave the hospital without a clue as to how to start the diet, where to get the foods, or how to adjust the diet to different situations (such as eating in restaurants).

If you've been used to eating a certain way all your life and are suddenly expected to change, you'll need to have a thorough understanding of how to make such changes. There may be a nutritionist at the hospital who can explain the diet in detail or your doctor may be able to recommend someone else who can do it.

## WHAT KIND OF EXERCISE SHOULD I BE GETTING?

Some people expect that they're going to be running 100-yard dashes up and down the stairs—down to the laundry room, up to the kitchen, up again to the kids' room, and back down again to the basement—as soon as they arrive home from the hospital. Sometimes it's nice to have the doctor tell you that you can't, in fact, go up and down stairs after surgery. After an episiotomy (done after a baby is delivered), for example, it's recommended that women refrain from climbing stairs for one to three weeks. Also, after undergoing treatment for certain cardiac problems, you may be advised to take some time off from excessive stresses and strains in order to let your heart develop exercise tolerance.

People tend to associate the word "exercise" with sit-ups and deep knee bends. But daily activities ranging from light housework to shoveling snow should also be considered exercise when recovering from surgery. Even driving a car can be too strenuous after some operations. Ask your doctor when you can return to these tasks.

In some cases, you may be required to carry out certain activities after leaving the hospital. For example, if you have been suffering intense pain from claudication (a blockage in the circulation, frequently in the lower extremities), the physician will usually tell you to do as much walking as possible to increase your circulation.

## SHOULD I BE FOLLOWING A SPECIAL EXERCISE PROGRAM?

Exercises can span the range of the entire muscular system. They can be as simple as a 100-foot daily walk or call for a jog of several miles. And they can be as esoteric and complicated as Kagel exercises, which involve tightening and relaxing the peroneal muscles of the groin— the muscles that control urination. When properly exercised, these muscles can prevent such conditions as stress incontinence, in which you lose urine upon coughing, laughing, or sneezing.

Ask your doctor what kind of exercise is best for you following your surgery.

## CAN SOMEONE EXPLAIN THIS EXERCISE REGIMEN TO ME IN DETAIL?

This question should be asked for the same reasons that you want a recommended diet thoroughly explained. If a doctor says, "You need to get out and walk," do you know just what he means? Does he mean a slow stroll around the block? Or a fast jog through the park? How many times a week? For how long at a time? You want detailed and specific instructions so that there's no doubt in your mind as to what you should (or should not) be doing.

## HOW MUCH REST SHOULD I BE GETTING?

You want to know to what extent rest is important to your recovery. After a bout with tuberculosis or some other overwhelming infection, for example, the body tends to need as much rest as possible. Exercise and activities are to be avoided so that the body can build up its strength and fight the infection. Rest is also effective for some back injuries, where exercise and activity can actually worsen the injury. In these instances, insufficient rest can cause a relapse or significantly slow your recovery.

Be sure you know how much rest is advised—and be sure to listen to the signals you get from your own body. Often they will tell you more than any doctor can.

## AFTER THE SURGERY IS OVER, WHO WILL SEND ME BILLS?

This is an excellent question to ask, because you will probably receive bills from a number of people with whom you will have had little or no direct contact.

The radiologist (the person who reads your x-rays) is one of these people. It's likely that you'll never meet the radiologist, since technicians perform the actual x-raying and the radiologist often only does the reading.

Technicians are employees of and are paid by the hospital. The radiologist is an M.D. who has gone through medical school, with an additional program in radiology, and is usually board certified. The radiologist will often be able to aid in a diagnosis based solely on what she sees in an x-ray.

Another person by whom you're liable to be billed is the pathologist. The pathologist is a medical doctor who has done a residency training program in the science of pathology.

Pathology is the laboratory study of disease and involves studying blood and tissue under a microscope. A forensic pathologist deals in legal pathology; for instance, he is called upon if a person dies in mysterious circumstances. The pathologist can estimate the time of death by studying the tissues. He also examines projectiles, such as bullets or glass, that might be involved in an accident, and he studies drug and alcohol levels. "Quincy," the popular TV series, featured a forensic pathologist.

With general surgery, pathologists evaluate tissue specimens removed during the procedure to see if any cancer is present or to study the nature of the tissue.

Thus you can expect to get bills from at least three people you may have seen, perhaps once, if ever: the radiologist, the pathologist, and the anesthesiologist.

You'll also get bills from your surgeon and from any consultants who are called in. Anytime a doctor comes in to examine you, you can ask, "Who are you? Will I be receiving a bill for this examination?"

## WHO IS THE RADIOLOGIST (THE PATHOLOGIST, THE ANES-THESIOLOGIST)? WHAT ARE THEIR NAMES? WHERE ARE THEIR OFFICES? WHAT ARE THEIR BILLING PROCEDURES?

Often you will receive separate bills from each of these doctors. They have separate offices and you have to deal with them on an individual basis. It's best to find out who they are while you're still in the hospital. That's much easier than trying to get this information after you've been discharged.

## DO I NEED TO SEE YOU AGAIN FOR A FOLLOW-UP VISIT?

The surgeon will want to see you for a follow-up exam to make sure that your recovery is going smoothly. She may need to remove stitches, bandages, or casts. Any questions you have about the outcome of the surgery and your present condition should be asked at this time.

## SHOULD I MAKE A FOLLOW-UP VISIT TO MY PRIMARY HEALTH CARE PHYSICIAN?

Your regular doctor will surely want to see you as a follow-up to your hospital stay. He'll want to see how the surgery went; he'll want to see how you're progressing in your recovery. And he'll want to determine what changes, if any, are necessary in your diet, activity, or medication.

# SMART QUESTIONS TO ASK AN ANESTHESIOLOGIST

Any time you have surgery done, major or minor, some kind of anesthetic will be used. An anesthetic is any substance that produces a loss of sensation, with or without loss of consciousness.

Not very long ago, whiskey was the most widely used anesthetic. Modern science has come a long way in a short time. The discovery of present-day anesthetics has allowed us greatly to expand our healing powers and our explorations of the human miracle.

As stated in the last section, however, anesthetics have by no means been perfected. There are risks involved, and you should have a thorough understanding of what those risks are before you consent to surgery.

Also covered in the last section was the fact that the anesthesiologist is directly responsible for your health

141

during and immediately following surgery. The anesthesiologist will probably come into your hospital room once before your surgery, ask you some questions, and evaluate your overall health and ability to undergo an operation. He will literally have your life in his hands, and yet he's someone you've barely met.

Not only will asking questions give you information about anesthesia, but doing so will also give you a chance to establish a relationship with the anesthesiologist. Your questions will remind him that you are a unique individual rather than the 8:00 a.m. mastectomy. They will make you both feel more human.

## WHAT ARE THE DIFFERENT KINDS OF ANESTHESIA?

The different kinds of anesthesia are regional, local, and general. General anesthesia involves putting the whole mental process in a cloud, desensitizing the whole body. It effects the brain, which, in turn, affects all the sensory organs.

Regional anesthetics affect only a particular region of the body. They are injected into a large nerve, which causes numbness in every area of the body that the nerve innervates. For example, a brachial block under the arm will numb most of the arm, from the upper arm down to the tips of the fingers.

Another regional block is the epidural (often used during labor to ease the pain), whereby the spinal cord below the third lumbar is numbed, causing most of the lower body to go to sleep.

Local anesthesics are injected into the soft tissue around the area where the surgeon plans to do the surgery. The average person is most familiar with local anesthesia as used during dental surgery, when Novocain is injected under the gum.

## DO I NEED TO HAVE GENERAL ANESTHESIA?

The anesthesiologist is responsible for determining which form of anesthesia will be used during surgery. Major surgery usually requires general anesthesia, but there are other types of surgery in which regional, or even local, anesthetics will suffice.

Ask the anesthesiologist to explain what type of anesthesia will be used and why. Find out if you have any options. Is this surgery ever done with a regional anesthetic rather than a general one? Under what circumstances? Which does the surgeon prefer? Which does the anesthesiologist recommend?

## IF I HAVE TO UNDERGO GENERAL ANESTHESIA, HOW AM I GOING TO FEEL WHEN I WAKE UP?

You may already have asked your surgeon just how you'll feel when you get out of surgery. It can't hurt to ask again. Remember, you're not only asking to get information. You want to establish a relationship with the anesthesiologist. Ask her to explain why anesthetics cause you to feel dizzy and nauseous. If you're undergoing regional or local anesthesia, ask her to explain the effects on the body and how you'll feel as the anesthetic wears off.

## WHAT ARE SOME OF THE COMPLICATIONS OF GENERAL ANESTHESIA?

When the anesthesiologist visits you before your operation, he'll ask you about your family history, any allergies you might have, and if you've ever had problems with anesthesia in the past.

In the majority of cases, there are no problems. If you've never had anesthesia before, however, there is no way of telling what your reaction will be. In rare instances, patients simply stop breathing under anesthesia, or they experience a sudden sharp rise in temperature and begin to have seizures. These instances do not occur often, but they do happen. The anesthesiologist can tell you what the statistics are and evaluate your potential for adverse reactions.

## WHAT ARE THE POSSIBLE COMPLICATIONS OF REGIONAL ANESTHESIA?

Occasionally, a patient experiences nerve injury and subsequent pain from the injection of the anesthestic. With epidurals, there is the possibility of respiratory suppression, or the inability to breathe, because the anesthestic makes its way up the spinal canal to the higher nerves of the chest, which makes breathing difficult. This complication is usually avoided if the patient is kept in a more vertical position.

## WHAT ARE THE POSSIBLE COMPLICATIONS OF LOCAL ANESTHESIA?

Adverse reactions to local anesthesia are infrequent. You could have an allergic reaction to the anesthetic, resulting in excessive itching, but this type of reaction tends to be mild and short-lived.

SECTION 10

# SMART QUESTIONS TO ASK ABOUT HOSPITAL PROCEDURES

You're scheduled for surgery tomorrow. You're nervous and want to get it over with. You go through the hospital door, stop, and look around you. You're not sure what to do. You hope you've brought everything you need; you're not thinking clearly. There are hospital personnel behind a desk, but they're paying no attention to you. People are coming and going all around you. You feel lost and afraid.

This is the experience of thousands of people as they enter a hospital, but it doesn't have to be your experience. There are many questions you can ask before you even get to the hospital—questions about admissions, about hospital policy, about all the procedures that go on there. All of these procedures, even the most basic, can seem mystifying and frightening—unless you ask questions.

This section contains sample questions in several different categories: choice of hospital, admissions procedures, recovery room procedures, your accommodations, and hospital personnel.

You'll never be completely free of fear and anxiety during your hospital stay. You can't be your own doctor or oversee your own operation. But you can take charge of your own education and attitude. The more you learn about the hospital, the less anxious you'll be. The less anxiety you have, the better are your chances of going in with a positive attitude and leaving with the promise of a speedy recovery.

## TO WHICH HOSPITAL DO YOU PLAN TO ADMIT ME?

The answer may be obvious—if there's only one hospital in the region. It may not be so obvious if your physician is associated with several hospitals. If you have a preference, now is the time to state it.

## WHICH WOULD BE THE BEST HOSPITAL FOR ME (PROVIDED THERE'S A CHOICE)?

Usually, the doctor who's going to be doing the surgery will choose the hospital at which he feels the most comfortable. If your surgeon is comfortable, you probably will be, too.

If you are not, you may have to choose another hospital—and another surgeon. For instance, if the hospital is in an area that's difficult for you and your family to get to, you may decide you'd rather not go there. If that's the only affiliation your surgeon has, you'll have to choose a different surgeon as well as a different hospital.

## DOES THIS HOSPITAL HAVE A GOOD REPUTATION?

This is an important question and you should use several different sources for your answer. Ask your primary health care physician's opinion. Ask people who have had surgery at this particular hospital. And, if you wish, check with your state or local health board or medical association. The quality of care you receive can vary greatly from hospital to hospital. Do as much research as you possibly can and don't make a decision based on one doctor's recommendation.

## WHAT TYPE OF HOSPITAL IS THIS?

What you're really asking here is: Is this a public, private, or university teaching hospital? One reason for asking is so you can check with your insurance company and make sure that all types of hospitals are covered.

## WHAT IS A PRIVATE HOSPITAL?

"Private" means that the hospital is a privately held corporation and is not publicly funded. It is usually a "for-profit" organization. Private hospitals are probably the best financed of any type of hospital. They tend to have new equipment and very friendly staffs. They are also the most expensive of all the hospitals.

## WHAT IS A PUBLIC HOSPITAL?

Public hospitals are usually financed by the cities or large metropolitan areas in which they are located. They are built specifically for the good of the people. The public hospital is like any other of the city's public works—it is there to provide a necessary service for the people of that area. The medical staffs in public hospitals tend to be very dedicated and hardworking.

There are other public hospitals that are located in smaller communities and are established to serve a large segment of the population. These hospitals may not be luxurious and may not have all of the latest equipment and the specialists to work with it, but to the people in the community there are things more important than having the best or the newest or the most expensive. It's not unusual for the nursing staff at a small community hospital to be taking care of their own relatives. There's a sense of family and individual care that you may not get in larger, more modern facilities.

## WHAT IS A TEACHING HOSPITAL?

The university teaching hospitals are a breed apart. Usually, being part of a large university, they are well funded. They have the most modern equipment and the medicine that is practiced in these institutes is always the most up-to-date. Optimal medical care is usually defined by what goes on at these university teaching hospitals.

The drawback of being in a teaching hospital, however, is that you tend to feel like a guinea pig in a vast experiment. In a sense, this is what you are, because the purpose of a teaching hospital is to teach medical students how to do their jobs. And they're using you to learn on.

I remember giving birth to my daughter Laura in a Long Island teaching hospital. It seemed as though every intern and resident on staff came in to look me over. I received a lot of attention, but very little rest and relaxation—the parade of doctors was continuous.

As Dr. Strauss explains, "When I was a third-year medical student at my university hospital, I was the first person to see the patients when they came into the hospital. I would ask them many, many questions and I would do a physical examination. The purpose of this was mostly for my own training in asking questions and conducting physical examinations.

"Next, a fourth-year medical student would come in. After this student finished her evaluation, she would present the case to the intern, who was a first-year resident.

"The first-year intern is also still learning, but has completed medical school and actually has an M.D. after his name. At this point, the patient usually thinks, 'I guess this must really be the doctor.'

"The intern asks all the pertinent questions and does another physical examination. He is, in fact, the front-line evaluator. He plans the treatment for the patient. The intern then presents the case to the senior resident (the boss of all the medical students and of the interns and residents who are under him), who evaluates the patient again.

"Finally, after all this, the senior resident must present the case to the attending physician. Frequently, it is the attending physician who admitted the patient to begin with.

"If the patient has a serious problem and doesn't have a sense of humor, the teaching hospital can be a very frustrating place. But the teaching hospital is a necessary entity. Where else can a doctor-in-training get the hands-on experience he or she needs?"

A teaching hospital can be a learning experience for the patient as well. If you're interested in your own body, and in medicine in general, you can learn along with the students. It can also be a difficult experience. You may not get as much rest, or privacy, as you would like. When you know how a teaching hospital works, and ask questions before you get there, you'll be prepared for all these interruptions.

## HOW THOROUGH ARE THE X-RAY AND DIAGNOSTIC LABORATORIES IN THIS HOSPITAL?

Some hospitals have a better reputation in this area than others. Your surgeon may have a feeling for how well tests are done at a particular hospital. Or friends who have been treated at this hospital may have had exposure to the laboratories and have opinions of their own. The more people you ask, the more objective an opinion you can form yourself.

## HOW FRIENDLY IS THE NURSING STAFF?

The people you come into contact with most often at the hospital are the nurses and the nursing staff. These people can make a big difference in the quality of your hospital stay. It doesn't take much asking around to find out "how friendly" a hospital's staff is. All you have to do is ask people who've been there and they'll tell you whether they had a good experience or a bad one. However, friendliness does not necessarily equal excellent care. Before you enter the hospital, inquire about the nurses' training, their degrees, the length of their shifts, etc.

## WHAT IS THE NURSE-TO-PATIENT RATIO?

This can be an important factor—especially if there is a shortage of nurses. If that's the case, not only do the nurses tend to be overworked (and less friendly), but they also tend to be under more stress (which could mean that they make more mistakes). And the last thing you want when you're in the hospital is to be worried that the staff doesn't seem to have the time or the proper concern for your health and well-being.

## DOES THE HOSPITAL HAVE A BROCHURE TO EXPLAIN SOME OF ITS POLICIES?

A lot of facilities do have brochures that explain hospital policies, what you can expect when you come to the hospital and who you can contact if there's a problem. This information is good for you to have, and also to pass on to family and friends.

## WHAT IS THE ADMISSIONS PROCEDURE AT THE HOSPITAL?

Patients often show up at the hospital feeling confused and disoriented because they haven't found out what they're supposed to do at the time of admission.

You need to know when to show up, exactly where to go (especially in a large hospital complex), and what to bring with you (identification, insurance forms, etc.).

## SHOULD I TALK TO ANYONE SPECIAL WHEN I GET TO THE HOSPITAL?

If you are to see someone specific in the department of admissions when you check in, you want to make sure you know exactly who it is and where you'll find him. You might even ask your physician to advise someone in the admitting office that you are expected at a certain time.

If this person is alerted to the fact that you're coming

to the hospital, and thus you have someone specific to ask for, you might speed up the admission procedure.

## HOW LONG DOES THE ADMISSION PROCESS USUALLY TAKE?

You should be prepared for a long wait, especially if the hospital is having an unexpectedly busy day. However, if you ask this question beforehand, you won't be surprised or upset if it takes an hour before you get past the desk and up to your room.

Check with your doctor (and with the hospital) to find out if there are any preadmission procedures that can be done to speed up the process. Sometimes paperwork can be taken care of ahead of time, especially where insurance is concerned.

## DO I NEED TO BRING ORDERS FROM THE DOCTOR?

If you are going to be admitted to a hospital, your physician will prepare a series of orders for you. You may be asked to bring the orders with you or they may be waiting for you at the nurses' station.

## WHAT KIND OF ORDERS HAVE YOU SET UP FOR ME?

Going into the hospital is always a nerve-racking experience, whether it's for minor surgery or an extensive stay. The more you know about what to expect while you're there, the less frightening the experience will be. If a nurse comes in to stick a very large needle in your arm, you won't be so scared if you know in advance that this is something the doctor has ordered.

You want to know if you can expect a lot of blood tests

or if you'll need x-rays, and why all these tests are being done. Sometimes it's just hospital policy and sometimes the tests are very specifically related to your surgery. The more you learn about what to expect once you get to the hospital, the more prepared you will be for the surgery and the easier your recovery period will be.

## SHOULD I HAVE A PRIVATE OR SEMIPRIVATE ROOM?

If you want complete privacy, you must make arrangements ahead of time. However, not all insurance companies will cover the cost of a private room, although some will if the physician orders it.

## WHAT ARE THE HOSPITAL VISITING HOURS? ARE THERE ANY RESTRICTIONS ABOUT WHO CAN VISIT?

This information can easily be obtained from the hospital. Some facilities restrict the number of people allowed to visit your room at any one time and many don't allow children under a certain age to visit patients (but will bend the rules under specific circumstances).

Some hospitals will allow a parent or a spouse to stay overnight. You can check this out by calling the hospital beforehand or asking the nurses when you arrive.

## WHAT SHOULD I BRING TO THE HOSPITAL WITH ME?

You want to know whether or not the hospital supplies sundries like toothbrushes and toothpaste. Most do, but it's good to know. You probably want to bring a bathrobe and slippers and perhaps a book or some magazines.

Don't have expensive jewelry, a lot of cash, or items of

sentimental value with you. Such things often get lost or stolen, especially in large metropolitan hospitals.

## WHAT'S GOING TO HAPPEN AFTER MY SURGERY, WHEN I'M IN THE RECOVERY ROOM?

Usually, nothing happens in the recovery room except recovery. Most people in the recovery room are not up to doing anything specific, like eating, drinking, or going to the bathroom.

You might not even be aware that you were ever in the recovery room. Barring any complications, you'll be returned to your room when your vital signs are stable. It's possible for you to sleep through the whole experience and not remember it at all.

## HOW LONG WILL I STAY IN THE RECOVERY ROOM AFTER SURGERY?

Some patients require a recovery room stay of only a half hour to an hour, while others may spend several hours. It depends on the type of surgery and the individual patient.

Complications sometimes develop while a patient is in the recovery room, necessitating a longer stay there or transferral to the intensive care unit for closer monitoring.

## CAN I HAVE VISITORS IN THE RECOVERY ROOM?

Visitors may be allowed in the recovery room, especially when the time there is prolonged for one reason or another. This decision often depends on the recovery room nurses and whether or not they're prepared to deal with anyone other than patients.

## WHAT ARE YOU CHECKING?

This is a question to ask anyone you deal with in the recovery room. Among the functions that are usually monitored are urinary output (how fast and how much you're urinating) and your vital signs (blood pressure, pulse, respiration, temperature). These are checked often, in emergency situations even every 5, 10, or 15 minutes. If you're awake and alert, there's no harm in asking what the readings are and why they're being taken.

## SHOULD I HAVE SOMEONE WAITING FOR ME IN MY ROOM?

When I had surgery a few years ago, I was so "spaced out" from the anesthetic that I had difficulty functioning by myself for 24 hours. It's a good thing my husband was there to give me a hand when I returned to my room.

This is an especially good question if there's a shortage of nurses or if the hospital is very busy.

## WHY DO THE NURSES COME IN SO OFTEN TO CHECK MY PULSE, TEMPERATURE, AND BLOOD PRESSURE?

This is usually standard procedure. These are your vital signs and they are checked at the beginning of each shift, more often if warrented.

## WHO ARE YOU? WHAT IS YOUR FUNCTION?

People walk in and out of your room all the time, and almost everybody wears a stethoscope. It's hard to know who's the doctor, who's the nurse, who's the orderly, who's the nurse's aide, who's the respiratory therapist, and so on.

You have a right to know who is in your room and what he or she plans to do there. You may want to ask some other questions, such as, "Did the doctor order you to be here?" "If so, why did the doctor order you to be here?" "What is it that you're doing to me?" "Why are you doing it?"

## WHAT ACTIVITIES WILL I BE ALLOWED WHEN I GET BACK TO MY ROOM?

Depending on the doctor's orders, you may or may not be allowed to get out of bed. You may only be allowed to go to the bathroom or you may be allowed to go anywhere you please. You don't want to do anything that will be bad for your health or add to your recovery time, so it's best to check with your doctor before you do anything.

## WHAT KIND OF FOOD AND BEVERAGES WILL I BE SERVED IN THE HOSPITAL?

If you've had knee surgery, your food intake probably will not be affected at all. Other kinds of surgery may require you to introduce solid foods gradually.

Dr. Strauss explains: "After surgery, diet is usually 'advanced as tolerated.' That's the lingo that we use, and it means we slowly advance the patient's diet to see how much he can eat and what kinds of food he can tolerate. We start off with clear liquids (if you hold the beverage up to the light, you can see the light through the liquid), which will be easily tolerated by your system. After clear liquids are tolerated, the patient is generally advanced to full liquids, that means those substances which are soft but not transparent, such as ice cream or prune juice.

"Following the full liquids, mechanical softs are allowed. These are substances that are easily chewed (so that people without teeth can eat them) and easily digested. They could include rice and potatoes and even chicken. After that, almost any foods can be tolerated (provided the patient is not being put on a restricted diet)."

It's better to know what you'll be allowed to eat, and when, so that you don't eat something you shouldn't.

## CAN I HAVE A BEDSIDE COMMODE?

The bedside commode is a portable potty chair that can be used in place right next to your bed. This can be more convenient than trying to use a bedpan, and yet it saves the discomfort of going all the way to the bathroom.

## AM I ALLOWED TO WATCH TELEVISION?

Usually this matter is decided among the patients in the room. Dr. Strauss adds, "I tell people they can watch TV as long as their roommate says it's okay, and as long as I can tolerate it when I'm in the room."

## DOES THE HOSPITAL PROVIDE THE TELEVISION SET OR DO I HAVE TO RENT IT?

Some hospitals have a television set in every room, and it is included in the cost of the room. In other hospitals, you have to pay for the privilege of watching television. The service is usually provided by an outside company, which will bill you separately for "television rental."

This is something that you can find out by calling the hospital before you're admitted or by reading the hospital brochure (if one is available).

## WILL I HAVE TELEPHONE PRIVILEGES?

Again, this varies from hospital to hospital. It may even vary from room to room. Most often, there is a telephone next to each bed and the costs of your calls are added to your hospital bill.

Some facilities allow only incoming calls and any outgoing calls must be made on the pay phones, unless special arrangements have been made. As with the television situation, check this out before you're admitted so you won't have any problems or surprises once you are in the hospital.

## WHY AM I BEING DISCHARGED?

When the doctor comes in and tells you it's time to be discharged, you might want to ask: "Why is it time to be discharged? Is it because I'm better? Or is it because my insurance runs out at a certain time and will no longer cover my stay?"

Believe it or not, hospitals are under tremendous pressure to get patients out quickly. Make sure that you're not kicked out of the hospital because of third-party (insurance) considerations before you're well.

## WHOM DO I CONTACT IF I HAVE A COMPLAINT?

If the hospital doesn't have a brochure, or if this information isn't included, this is an important question for you to ask. Frequently, there is an ombudsman—a patient advocate who is a troubleshooter. This person is a hospital employee.

## WHEN I LEAVE THE HOSPITAL, CAN I DONATE SOME OF MY FLOWERS TO PEOPLE WHO HAVE NONE?

I hope that you are fortunate enough to have family and friends who care about you. If that's true, you might find that you are overwhelmed by the amount of flowers and balloon bouquets you receive during your hospital stay. You might even decide that you don't have enough room at home for all of these lovely gifts.

There are people in the hospital who have no visitors, receive no calls or cards, and have nothing to brighten up their rooms. These people are often appreciative of any small gesture.

Check with the nurses to see if anyone on your floor is in that situation. You may decide to visit this patient and deliver the flowers personally.

# SECTION 11

## SMART QUESTIONS TO ASK WHEN YOU'RE PLANNING TO TRAVEL

You're planning a trip. You've been very careful to make sure you have everything you need. You have clothes for sightseeing and clothes for fancy restaurants. You have bathing suits and extra sweaters. You have your passport and your traveler's checks.

You've made a list, and you've gone over it thoroughly. You've checked everything—except your health.

What do you know about the country you're visiting? What happens if you get sick in a foreign country? What do you do about the medication you're taking now? What if you run out?

Don't wait until you're flying across the ocean to think of these things. Ask questions before you leave. I'm sure you'll think of more questions than are listed here. Ask your doctor, ask your travel agent, ask friends who've already traveled to the country you're about to visit. Get all the information you can before you leave. Nothing makes a better traveling companion than peace of mind!

## I'M TRAVELING TO ANOTHER STATE (OR COUNTRY). DO YOU KNOW A DOCTOR I COULD CALL ON IN AN EMERGENCY?

If you have a medical condition such as diabetes, a heart problem, or asthma, you probably want to be prepared whenever you travel. Even if you're perfectly healthy, it's always good to know of someone you can contact in an emergency.

Your doctor may know someone in the state or city you're planning to visit. Doctors often belong to medical associations and attend conventions at which they meet colleagues from other areas of the country or from abroad.

## WHAT KINDS OF HEALTH PROBLEMS CAN I EXPECT TO RUN INTO ON TRAVELS ABROAD?

Some of these health problems are rather well known, such as traveler's diarrhea, which is ubiquitous in certain parts of Mexico, or malaria in some third world countries. It's best to be prepared. Do your own research: read books about the country and try to find people who've been there so they can give you a first-hand account.

## WHAT KIND OF PREVENTATIVE HEALTH MEASURES CAN I TAKE BEFORE MY TRIP?

This really depends on where you're going. There are certain ports of the world where it's strongly recommended that potential visitors be immunized against certain diseases before they leave the United States. For example, yellow fever is still endemic in several areas and it's a good idea to be immunized against it before you go to those countries. Ask your doctor, and you can also check with the tourist board of the country you're planning to visit to see what it recommends.

## WHAT CAN I DO WHILE TRAVELING TO STAY AS HEALTHY AS POSSIBLE?

In a lot of areas, hygiene is important. Your doctor may be able to describe some of the hygiene problems of a particular area. There are preventative measures you can take, such as drinking only bottled beverages and being aware of the fact that fruits and vegetables generally have a high risk of transmitting infectious disease.

## WHERE WOULD YOU RECOMMEND I GO IF I SHOULD FEEL SICK?

Your doctor may or may not know the answer to this question. Ask your travel agent to find the names and addresses of doctors in the areas in which you'll be traveling.

Of course, if you're ill, you want to be able to communicate with the doctors. If you don't understand the language of an area, find out if there's a hospital there where English is spoken or a doctor who speaks English. Once again, your travel agent may be able to provide you with this information. Or perhaps you can find out from the hotel at which you will be staying.

"I've had patients from foreign countries who are unable to speak English," adds Dr. Strauss. "In order to provide such a patient with the proper health care, it was necessary to locate a translator, and this took some time. If you're traveling to a country where you don't speak the language, it might be helpful to know where translators can be found in the event of an emergency."

## SHOULD I TAKE MY MEDICINE WITH ME ON MY TRIP?

You should always take your regular medicines with you on your trips. In fact, you should make sure that you have an adequate supply before you leave.

## COULD YOU GIVE ME ENOUGH TO LAST ME UNTIL I GET BACK?

You might find it very difficult to get a prescription in another language, and it could take a long time to have new medication mailed or wired to you overseas. If you think there's any chance that you might run out before you return, ask your doctor to supply you with the proper amount.

It's also a good idea to take along more than you need and to keep the medication in two separate containers. That way, if one container is lost or damaged, you'll still have medication safely stored somewhere else.

## IS THERE ANY SPECIAL WAY I SHOULD CARRY OR STORE MY MEDICINE?

Most medicines are easily stored in the standard pill bottle. If you're going to run into extreme weather conditions, however, this is an important question to ask. Capsules, for example, can melt and decompose in excessive humidity and heat. Liquids can congeal and, in some instances, solidify. Ask your physician how best to care for your medication. Some of this information can also be obtained from the pharmacist.

## WILL MY INSURANCE COVER MEDICAL BILLS FROM A FOREIGN COUNTRY?

This is something you will need to check with your individual insurance company and it should be done before you go on your trip.

# CONCLUSION

# TEN KEY POINTS CONCERNING YOU, YOUR HEALTH, AND YOUR DOCTOR

## 1. TAKE RESPONSIBILITY FOR YOUR OWN HEALTH AND WELL-BEING.

This is something you can and must, do. It doesn't mean that you have to become your own doctor. It does mean you have to make informed choices about the doctors you consult, the hospitals you go to, and the treatments and medications you take.

## 2. STAND UP FOR YOUR RIGHT TO ASK QUESTIONS.

You have to be persistent. A doctor may not want, or be prepared, to answer all your questions, but you must insist. If she says she is too busy, ask when she'll be free and make an appointment to call her.

## 3. BE AWARE THAT THE ONLY WAY TO GET THE INFORMATION YOU NEED IS BY ASKING QUESTIONS.

167

Don't be afraid to admit you don't know. Great inventions and scientific discoveries were made by people who "didn't know." They admitted to the world that they didn't have all the answers. Then they asked questions, questions, and more questions, until they found the answers they needed.

### 4. DISCOVER YOUR OPTIONS.

Options give you control over any situation. Never do anything (or refrain from doing anything) just because the doctor said so. Find out what your choices are and then make your decision.

### 5. ACCEPT THAT KNOWLEDGE REDUCES FEAR AND ANXIETY.

It's not what we know that scares us, it's what we don't know. Recovering from illness takes all the strength you have. You don't want to waste your energy on imaginary concerns.

### 6. NEVER ASSUME.

Don't assume that you have all the information you need. A doctor may have given similar instructions to 2,000 other people—but forget to give you one vital piece of information. Don't assume something is okay just because the doctor gave it to you, like my friend who became addicted to pills because she assumed the doctor wouldn't give her anything potentially harmful. Think about what you're doing, and make the doctor think as well!

### 7. DON'T ACCEPT AN EASY ANSWER. PROBE AND CLARIFY.

Little children do this automatically. Answer a question and they'll come back with a "Why?" every time. You should do the same. You want to be absolutely sure you understand everything that's going on with your body, your health.

## 8. REALIZE THAT A DOCTOR IS JUST A HUMAN BEING.

No matter how intimidating she may seem, a doctor really is just a human being. That means she can make human mistakes. She can also be warm, sympathetic, and understanding. Let her know what you need and how she can help you.

## 9. BUILD A ONE-ON-ONE RELATIONSHIP WITH YOUR DOCTOR.

You don't have to become best friends. But asking questions sets up an immediate rapport with the doctor. The doctor's attitudes, as well as his answers, will give you important clues about his background and personality.

Your questioning attitude lets him know that you're special, and that you intend to take part in the process of maintaining your health. Remember that the doctor and the patient must work together. The ideal doctor/patient relationship is one in which both parties share the responsibility for proper health care.

## 10. ASK SMART QUESTIONS. ASK SMART QUESTIONS. ASK MORE SMART QUESTIONS.

If you want to know more about Dorothy Leeds' speeches, seminars, and audiocassette programs, please call or write to:

Dorothy Leeds, President
Organizational Technologies Inc.
800 West End Avenue Suite 10A
New York, NY 10025
(212) 864-2424
(800) 423-1169

Her Positive Action Cassette Learning Programs are the following:

*Smart Questions: The Key to Sales Success.* This unique and proven program will help you improve your questions to solve the mystery of the decision-making process, uncover the right information in the right way at the right time, practice sure-fire ways to answer objections, and close the sale.

*PowerSpeak: The Complete Guide to Persuasive Public Speaking and Presenting.* You can easily become a powerful and persuasive presenter by following Dorothy Leeds' proven PowerSpeak method.

*The Motivational Manager: How to Get Top Performance from Your Staff.* Being an excellent manager is the best way to get ahead. With this motivational program you will discover your strengths and weaknesses, how to hire, coach, train, motivate, and lots more.

*People Reading: Strategies for Engineering Better Relationships in Business.* Gain a huge career advantage by influencing others and achieving results through reading the unique differences in people.

# INDEX

## A

Abnormal behavior, 116

Accomodations, hospital, 146, 153-154, 156-158

Activities, postoperative, 156

Acupuncture, 12

Acute condition, 57

Addiction, vs. dependency, 84

Addiction potential, 85

Admission procedures, 146, 151-152

AIDS, risk of contracting, 45

Alcoholism, treatments for, 71

Allergies, 59; children's, 113; as genetic, 62; predisposition to, 63

Alopath, 21

Alternative treatments, 70-71, 98; exercise as, 82; to surgery, 124-125

Altzheimer's disease, 59

Amblyopia, 115

American College of Oncologists, 102

American College of Pediatricians, 110

American College of Radiologists, 102

American Medical Association (AMA), 10

Amniocentesis, 104

Amoxicillin, 78

Anesthesia: kinds of, 142; risks of, 131. *See also* Anesthetics

Anesthesiologist: questions concerning, 141-144; responsibility of, 141-142; role of in surgery, 130. *See also* Nurse anethetist

Anesthetics, during delivery, 105-106; during surgery, 130

Antabuse (disulfiran), 71

Antibiotics, 72

Appointments, missed, 35

Assignment, accepting, 32-34

Asthma, 59-60

Attending physician, 149